Menstruation and Menopause

Alfred · A · Knopf · New York · 1976

Menstruation and Menopause

The Physiology and Psychology, the Myth and the Reality

by PAULA WEIDEGER

THIS IS A BORZOI BOOK
PUBLISHED BY ALFRED A. KNOPF, INC.

Grateful acknowledgment is made to the following for permission to reprint previously published material:

Bill Barnes: For an excerpt from "The Resemblance Between a Violin Case and a Coffin" by Tennessee Williams. Copyright 1950 by Tennessee Williams.

John Cushman Associates, Inc.: For an excerpt from *The Summer Before the Dark* by Doris Lessing. Copyright © 1973 by Doris Lessing. Originally published by Alfred A. Knopf, Inc.

Macmillan Publishing Co., Inc.: For an excerpt from *Symbolic Wounds* by Bruno Bettelheim. Copyright © 1962 by The Free Press of Glencoe, Inc.

William Morrow & Company, Inc.: For an excerpt from *Male and Female* by Margaret Mead. Copyright 1949, 1955 by Margaret Mead; and for an excerpt from *Sex and Temperament* by Margaret Mead. Copyright 1935 by Margaret Mead.

S. G. Phillips, Inc./Publisher: For an excerpt from *The New Golden Bough* by James Frazer, edited by Theodore Gaster. Copyright © 1959 by Criterion Books, Inc.

G. P. Putnam's Sons: For excerpts from *Woman's Mysteries* by M. Esther Harding. Copyright © 1971 by C. G. Jung Foundation for Analytical Psychology.

Library of Congress Cataloging in Publication Data
Weideger, Paula.
Menstruation and menopause.

Bibliography: p.
Includes index.
1. Menstruation.   2. Menstruation disorders.   3. Menopause.
4. Menstruation (in religion, folklore, etc.)   I. Title.
RG161.W44 1976   612.6'63   75–8262
ISBN 0–394–49647–7

Manufactured in the United States of America
First Edition

To Lillian Topper Weideger
and to the memory
of Michael Weideger

Contents

Illustrations

Acknowledgments

Hundreds of women contributed to this book and I thank all of them for answering the menstrual questionnaire and for their encouragement, and I thank the editors at *Ms.* magazine for giving me the space to announce that the questionnaire was available to all who might be interested in sharing their opinions and experiences. I also wish to thank all the women and men who provided me with and directed me toward research materials and pertinent literature, as well as Holly Canteen and Frieda Schutze, who translated portions of Ploss and Bartles from the German. (To the person who removed Volume I of the English translation of Ploss and Bartles from the New York Public Library, please return it *now*.) My thanks to the Macdowell Colony, where part of this book was written.

I am indebted to the late Hal Scharlatt—without his faith and commitment this book could not have existed.

My special thanks and appreciation to Vicky Wilson for her support from the very beginning to the end of this book, and for all the hard work and editorial skill she has applied to it.

Menstruation and Menopause

1

Veils and Variability

During the past few years women have been actively seeking knowledge about the female body and female experience—from the inside out. No longer content to be told what woman's experience *ought* to be, we are beginning to find out what it is. One of the results of this search is the growing awareness that we share a breadth of experience and that there is commonality in our differences. Through this process of sharing, a sense of community, rather than confusion, is being developed. The same result can be gained by sharing knowledge about the experiences of menstruation and menopause. Variation need not be a synonym for chaos.

Sharing of and respect for the experiences of menstruation and menopause can make an enormous and beneficial difference in women's lives. Although there are groups of women among whom these issues have been discussed, the majority of women have not yet participated. The silence about menstruation and menopause has blurred communication between mother and daughter, teacher and pupil, sister and sister. These events are a basic element in every woman's life, yet they remain veiled in silence.

Silence exists for two reasons: women have been ashamed of menstruation, and menopause and menstruating woman are taboo. The taboo of menstruation, of which menopause partakes, includes the precept that women shall keep these experiences hidden. When we are taught that something has to be hidden, we naturally believe that it contains an element that is not acceptable to other people. If menstruation were considered "clean," and menopause "decent," everyone would freely admit to their existence. We are ashamed of menstruation and menopause, we are taught to hide all evidence of their existence, and we have come to believe there is something in these experiences that is "wrong." This belief is reflected in our language—we don't call these events directly by name.

Menstruating woman has the "curse," "falls off the roof," "flies the Baker flag," "rides the rag," or is "unwell." To use more neutral words, she may have a "period" or a "visit from a friend." (Depending on the geographic area in which she lives, this friend may go by the name of Charlie or George.) At menopause she "goes through the changes," experiences the "change of life" or, as Virginia Woolf called it, the "T[ime] of L[ife]."

Having taught several women's health courses I knew before I began this book that once the subjects of menstruation and menopause are openly discussed, euphemism vanishes and a great variety of personal experiences and viewpoints begins to emerge. With this in mind, I prepared a questionnaire* to which 558 women replied.

One of the women who responded to the questionnaire pointed out that even the supposedly technical terms are themselves euphemisms. *Menstruation* is from the Latin for "monthly," *catamenia*, from the Greek "monthly," and *menopause* is also derived from the Greek, meaning "cessation of the month." All of the terms are tinged with our feelings of shame. Perhaps women will create a new terminology as we redefine the nature, as well as the meaning, of female experience.

The replies to the questionnaire make it obvious that while all women share the experiences of menstruation and menopause, there is no uniform assessment of the nature or meaning of these events. Here is a sample of their comments:

It [menstruation] makes me very much aware of the fact that I am a woman, and that's something very important to me. . . . It's also a link to other women. I actually enjoy having my period. I feel like I've been cleaned out inside. (M.P.W.)

The menstrual cycle has become such a part of my life by now, I don't want to change it. It is part of being a woman, which I am proud to be. (M.C.B.)

* The menstrual questionnaire is reproduced in the Appendix, along with a general description of the group that responded. An analysis of responses appears in appropriate sections of this book; the individuals' answers when quoted are indicated by their initials within parentheses.

I really like it. It's difficult to explain, but it's the same way I like the changing of the seasons. I guess the monthly cycles are "earthy" and symbolic to me. (R.J.C.)

Menopause, it's the best form of birth control. Face it graciously and brag about it. It's great. (S.F.)

and . . .

It's a pain—literally and figuratively. (V.M.)

During the time I was menstruating, which was from age eleven to age fifty-three, naturally I would have preferred no menstrual flow. (M.W.R.)

Menstruation is a pain in the vagina. (S.B.P.)

Menopause, can I get through it without collapse? Men don't have that damned inconvenience and discomfort. God must have been a man—a woman would have done a better job on women's bodies. (B.B.W.)

Women who enjoy menstruation and welcome menopause are no more peculiar than those who find menstruation a "pain" and menopause a frightening specter. As soon as women express their opinions, the laws of common knowledge collapse. The menstrual or menopausal experience of one woman need not—does not—hold true for another. The common views that menstruation and menopause are monoliths must be put aside, along with the prevailing opinion that they are distinctly negative experiences. It is time for an uncommon look at these cycles of life.

The uncommon view of menstruation and menopause begins with a new law: *Variation is the rule.*[1] Of course, there are facts about these states that apply to all women, but the exceptions and variations make up the far more abundant source of useful information. In every instance in which uniformity of experience is supposed to exist, a new look will uncover variation. We've already learned that this is true of women's attitudes toward menstruation and menopause. Another generality suggests that menstruation is valued solely as the bellwether of fertility.

Many women who are not interested in having more children, or in having children at all, continue to have interest in and positive feeling toward their menstrual cycles. Many women who are menopausal are happy to have fertility end and do not pine for the loss of its sign. I recently attended a concert where a song was sung that expressed good feelings about menstruation without a word about fertility. It was cheered by the audience—all of whom were women.

For some women, the menstrual cycle is not part of awareness, but the function of menstrual flow as a bellwether of fertility is most important. Whenever a woman fails to use contraceptives or suspects that her method of contraception has failed her, the sight of menstrual blood provokes a feeling that is a mixture of joy and relief. The woman who has been trying to conceive may find menstrual flow cause for feelings of disappointment and sorrow.

There is as much variance in the physical aspects of menstruation and menopause as there is in attitudes about them. The signs of menopause and their intensity differ from one woman to the next, as do manifestations of the menstrual cycle such as length of cycle and amount of flow. In each category there is a range of experience that is labeled normal. (The limits of the normal range are described in detail in the following chapter.)

Just as there is variation between individuals, there is variation across age groups. For example, the majority of adolescents *and* the majority of women approaching menopause have cycles in which there is no ovulation, while most women in the 20–40 age group have menstruation without ovulation only once or twice a year. The range of experience that is normal is not fixed throughout woman's life but changes as a function of her stage of life. You may acquire knowledge about the normal range of menstruation for members of your age group only to find that five years later your ideas are inapplicable.

So much variation may seem confusing. The experiences of menstruation and menopause are not intrinsically confusing, nor are they too complex to be learned by every woman. The confusion occurs because we have not been taught about these processes and have haphazardly absorbed information from the school of common knowledge. Because our education has been so poor, we start our mature lives with misconceptions that need constant amending. In fact, we would be better off to forget everything we thought we "knew," neglect amendment, and begin again.

As women, we are beginning to appreciate and respect both our similarities and our differences. And we are struggling to have what we know about female experience respected by others. The knowledge which has come from these struggles has particular application to menstruation and menopause. A constant reassessment of our assumptions is needed, and this is perhaps most obvious in relation to the treatment of problems associated with each state. (The most common of these problems and their possible causes and cures are discussed in detail in chapter 3.)

There is no one cause for a given difficulty with menstruation or menopause, and no one treatment which is successful or even appropriate for a given problem. Furthermore, there are not two separate categories of problem—the legitimate and the bastard. Many of us assume that our particular problems are legitimate but other people's may be somewhat questionable. This is one of the assumptions that needs re-examination. Women who do not have menstrual pain, for example, may think that those who do are manufacturing cramps in order to get sympathy or as an excuse to avoid some responsibility. In fact, this is sometimes true, but it is hardly the most likely explanation, nor is it reasonable to apply it prejudicially to another woman. The *absence* of a particular problem with menstruation or menopause is not the mark of a woman's moral superiority, nor is the presence of symptoms* de facto evidence of moral infirmity. Freedom from cramps (or any other menstrual or menopausal symptom) is not a sign of virtue.

Once women begin to consider the experiences of menstruation and menopause as legitimate parts of their lives and remove the moral judgments applied to those who have particular problems with these cycles of life, many things will change. Most obviously, women with problems will be encouraged to seek successful treatment.

In the matter of cramping, for example, one woman might find that exercise cures her, another will be helped by a well-timed shot of whiskey, and a third will find relief through an improved diet. (Menstrual pain is discussed in chapter 3, along with a list of remedies supplied by the women who answered the questionnaire.) The woman for whom nonmedical methods have failed may consult a physician. Once she comes to respect her problem and is supported by her peers, she will be more open to a discussion of the possible causes and treatments for her condition. If the physician similarly respects her problem, careful diagnosis will be made and treatment tried until success or relief of symptoms occurs. If the physician does not respect the problem, if he assumes an aura of moral superiority, frustration and confusion will result for the patient. He† may take the position

---

* The use of the word "symptom" in no way implies that menstruation or menopause are diseases or that the problems associated with them are indications of disease.

† The male personal pronoun is appropriate when talking about gynecologists, since in the U.S. 97% of the members of this group are men. Their problems, as well as our problems with them, are discussed in chapter 6.

that there ought to be one cause and one cure. If that cure fails, he may throw up his hands and blame the failure on his "intractable" patient.

Thus far neither doctor nor patient respects the experiences of menstruation and menopause. While Western women do not walk about in the drapery of Purdah, the veils of secrecy, shame, and disrespect similarly constrict the female personality. The unknown and hidden aspects of woman's life are sometimes described as the riddle of female identity and sometimes derided as the soiled evidence of corruption.

If in our use of language we obscure menstruation and menopause, in our actions we go to far greater lengths to hide the evidence. And the message of our actions is far more potent.

My mother bought me a box of Kotex and a belt and said, "Once a month you're going to be sick, here's where I'll put this stuff when you need it." . . . She opened a drawer and stuck it in. I was left stunned. When I started my period, the first three days or so I flowed very slowly and it was brownish. I didn't know that I had started and was afraid to ask my mom or anyone. I don't know how long (it seemed like years) that I went on not knowing what was going on with my body and sticking toilet paper in my underpants. It was really a traumatic experience for me.

It must have taken six months for me to feel free enough to ask my mom to buy some Kotex. It was okay during the week because I could buy it in the nickel machine but what a time I had on weekends. I only wish my mother would have remembered and replaced a new box from time to time! (M.R.C.)

The need to hide the evidence may become less intense with time but doesn't magically disappear with age and the repeated experience of menstruation, nor does it depend on unpleasant early experience to feed its continuity:

Menstruation's onset was not a traumatic experience for me, and so I have been spared that bewilderment or embarrassment. . . . Curiously, however, I still sometimes have twinges of uneasiness when purchasing tampons myself from a male clerk, accustomed as I am to the action. This does not stem from any lewd glances or speech on their part; it is some long-lasting reluctance within myself to announce my physical condition to the world, or to some male I do not know. (A.M.S.)

I have vivid memories of my teen-age walks from the store to my house burdened with an enormous box of napkins and an overwhelming feeling of humiliation. Never mind that the box was inside a brown paper bag, I was convinced that the whole neighborhood knew what it contained. The thought that the secret was out was enough to make me walk furtively while I fought back the blush of shame.

After more than two hundred cycles I no longer feel intense shame when purchasing supplies. (Although I suspect the blessedly small size of tampon cartons has been a source of relief.) For a couple of years I have bought tampons at a stationery store around the corner from my apartment. One day, the woman who owns the store handed me my change and remarked that we seem to get our periods at the same time. I looked up and smiled and realized that, in all the years since my teens, I had been wearing emotional armor whenever I bought tampons. When the woman in the stationery store made her remark, the armor was gone and in the moment it left me, I realized for the first time that it had existed.

Still, shame does linger on. In my case, it takes the form of feeling guilty about *any* emotion that I can definitely attribute to the menstrual cycle. Premenstrual tension, irritability, bursts of energy, and even increased sexual desire all seem not quite acceptable once I identify their connection to the menstrual cycle. It is as though the relationship between any state of feeling and menstruation proves that the feeling is not quite "real," not part of my "real self."

When I refuse to respect a feeling simply because I associate it with menstruation, I am in effect saying I don't want a self of which I am ashamed. Rather than *feel* shame, I deny these feelings. I may not feel ashamed, but I have chosen to deny *myself*. Once examined, this trade-off is no longer acceptable.

The sense of shame about menstruation is instilled as soon as menstruation begins. From the time of menarche, a girl learns to be ashamed of her body; she is told it limits her freedom, just because of the way it naturally functions. This shame continues throughout her life and is experienced into menopause. Any sign that menopause exists, for example, is as much a source of shame for a mature woman as the signs of menstruation are for a younger woman.

There are many ways in which the lesson of shame is taught, and it has great impact because little else is taught. Education about the biological, practical, and psychological aspects of menstruation and menopause is either lacking or superficial. Where there is a vacuum, there is plenty of folklore to fill it: "Hide menstruation, don't go swimming or wash your hair, or take baths or touch plants. And menopause . . . well you know that women go crazy then and lose all interest in sex . . ." These are some of the rumors whispered to young girls. How are they to learn to be proud to be a woman? How is the grown woman going to develop a feeling of pride in herself?

Poor education and the rumors that take up the slack, however, are not the first causes of the shame associated with menstruation and menopause. Education reflects an environment filled with the beliefs that foster shame and secrecy. This is the climate in which common knowledge thrives and the climate in which it is acceptable for men to take the moods of menstruating or menopausal women with especial casualness.

Sometimes if I am in a bad mood, my husband will not take me seriously if I am close to my period. He felt if it was "that time of the month" any complaints I had were only periodic. A few weeks ago I told him that until I am fifty-five he will have taken me seriously only half the time. After that he will blame it on menopause. Only after I am sixty-five will he take all my moods seriously. He said I had a legitimate gripe, so only time will tell if he's truly changed. (D.M.M.)

In chapters 7, 8, and 9 the ways in which menstruation and menopause influence female behavior are investigated. To say that the cycles influence behavior, however, is not to say that these changes of feeling are less real or valid than those unrelated to cyclicity. Since I am guilty of this confusion, I well know that logic is not synonymous with common knowledge. Too many of us have inherited the beliefs that menstruation and menopause are not really part of woman's life and that the feelings stemming from either state are not as "real" as our other feelings.

The denial of menstrual and menopausal realities, whether by women or by men, is part of the taboo of menstruation. For thousands of years, menstruating woman has been taboo. Like *any* object of taboo, she has been considered a source of danger. Historically, the pregnant woman and the woman in childbirth were also objects of taboo:

> The misfortunes brought about by pregnancy and childbirth parallel those of menstruation. Among the Indians of Costa Rica, a woman pregnant for the first time infects the whole neighborhood. . . . Cape Town Bantu males believe that looking upon a lying-in woman will result in their being killed in battle. Some Brazilian Indians are sure

that if the woman is not out of the house during childbirth weapons will lose their powers.[2]

In our culture the taboos of pregnancy and childbirth have disappeared. Indeed, now the father is often eager to be present at the delivery. While these taboos have dissipated, the menstrual taboo retains its age-old powers. "For man, menstruous woman is taboo. . . . The menstruation taboo is the most virulent of all taboos."[3] (Examples of the practices associated with the menstrual taboo are given throughout this book; the origins of the taboo are discussed in chapter 4.)

When a person is believed to harbor a power that may be dangerous to the group, controls are initiated in order to limit and contain this power. These controls form the rules of taboo. The powerful individual is tabooed. As long as everyone in the group (including the person of power) conforms to certain rules of behavior, that is, as long as the taboo is honored, the tabooed person's power is not discharged and the safety of the group remains unthreatened.

If the rules are broken, the power is unleashed and may fall upon anyone, but it is most likely to come to the person or people who have broken the regulations. In the case of menstruation, men and women are expected to obey the laws of the menstrual taboo; and if these laws are broken by a man, it is believed that his punishment (whatever it may be in a given culture or circumstance) results from the unleashed, terrible powers that dwell within menstruating woman at every moment. It is with some curiosity that we note that should menstruating woman herself break the taboo, little if any harm befalls her—women evidently have auto-immunity. However, should she break the taboo, the entire community or any of the male individuals within it may suffer grave harm.

Power . . . Taboo . . . Danger. These words (and the concepts behind them) appear to be far removed from the daily experience of menstruating and menopausal women in our culture. What woman in our culture will believe that men are afraid of her when she's menstruating or that men experience great relief when women reach menopause because the source of their fears has been removed? Not many of us will find the suggestion plausible. It is my purpose, however, to demonstrate that the menstrual taboo is still active because men still perceive in menstruating women the presence of a great and dangerous power.

One of the reasons why men do not directly experience the feeling

of fear in the presence of menstruating women is that we so completely hide menstruation. The taboo tells us that menstruation must
be hidden, we feel ashamed of menstruation and menopause as a
result, and by acting upon shame, we reinforce the taboo. Modern-day
women are not required to live in menstrual huts; modern-day men
are able to have menstruating women cook for them and wash their
dishes *because* women have so conscientiously and completely internalized the assumptions underlying the taboo. It is as though we have
constructed menstrual huts around our hearts and minds—and the
building blocks of these huts are shame and guilt.

If, and when, women break through shame and guilt, the walls of
the huts will collapse. This will be the time when male feelings of
danger and the anxiety it evokes may be more apparent.

*I went to visit a friend on the Lower East Side of New York. His
apartment was a disgusting mess—plaster falling from the walls and
ceiling, furniture broken down, dirty dishes all over, etc. He said a Zen
prayer for killing a living thing before squashing a two-inch roach with
his shoe.*

*Since the bathroom was out in the hall, I squatted down behind
some junk in the apartment, and started to change my tampon. When
he saw what I was doing, he became hysterical and ranted the rest of
the night about "uncleanliness" and how "unclean" women should
be segregated like in primitive tribes. The menstrual taboo is alive and
sick in modern society.* (M.G.)

Few women are able to break through the constraints applied to
menstruation and menopause. And unlike the woman in the story
quoted above, who was not ashamed, most of us will never know if
we would receive the same reaction in a similar situation. I suspect
many of us, however, believe his response would be often echoed. Our
conviction that men would act this way further reinforces the feeling
of shame we have learned since childhood, and the circle remains unbroken.

The fear of men's negative responses to menstruation and menopause is certainly not only in our minds. Not long ago, an outraged
audience responded to a television show in which menstruation was
mentioned. The writers of the Archie Bunker program, famous as a
forum in which many social taboos are trampled, received negative
letters following the episode in which menstruation was mentioned.
In fact, there was more mail than they had in response to any other
segment in the series.

As I worked on this book I naturally talked to many women and men about menstruation and menopause. A book in progress can function as an intermediary object in much the same way a camera separates the photographer from his subject. With a book in between, the power of the menstrual taboo remained safely within the bodies of menstruating women and the subject could be discussed rather openly, the words "menstruation" and "menopause" used freely. However, as soon as the subject was safely opened, people began to question the wisdom of keeping it open. Because some of these questions concern the purpose of this book, because they question the possible results of taking an uncommon look at menstruation and menopause, they require a detailed reply.

A committed misogynist will use any example of women's "weakness" to bolster his prejudice. He already uses the very existence of menstruation and menopause to "prove" that woman is unpredictable and unfit for positions of trust and responsibility. Of late, misogynists are called "male chauvinists," and their opinions "sexist." Sexism is pitted against feminism. Some of my colleagues expressed the fear that the information contained in this book might be used to raise the question: "Wouldn't it be better to keep silent about menstruation and menopause rather than risk adding ammunition to the sexist arsenal?"

Our silence sustains the menstrual taboo and keeps women in our present place of shamed hiding. So far this has not deterred misogynists, but it has limited women's self-knowledge and helped to create the situation in which we find ourselves today—subject to the prevailing male definition of women. The more we learn about ourselves, the more we will become ourselves. We cannot prevent men who need to keep "woman in her place" from using information about menstruation and menopause as it becomes available. We might have to continue to battle with men who use these tactics, but by speaking freely women will have gained definition and substance. When we are rid of menstrual shame and can work to change the attitudes toward menstruation and menopause, we will no longer be targets vulnerable to such attack.

Some of the women who questioned the value of re-examining menstruation and menopause felt that all that is necessary are a few biological facts: the heart pumps blood, nails grow, ears take in sound—and the reproductive system goes through its cycle. Menstruation and menopause are simple, biological events; to say more is to make too much of a small thing. Certainly, menstruation and menopause are biological events, but they are neither simple nor narrow in scope. The ramifications of the cycle of female sex hormone production take us beyond the realm of the biochemical and physiological. Menstruation and menopause are part of our emotional and social experience as well. For this reason I have incorporated the research of psychologists, sociologists, and anthropologists, and the shared experiences of many women, as an integral part of my text.*

Some men expressed concern about the implications of this book, believing that it might diminish the "feminine mystery" which they felt was central to art. Their perception of woman and her role in art is faithfully described in the following passage:

> Some days he was so blind to them he couldn't make out any resemblances to living forms at all on the canvases. But he knew they were women, like other women, and the endless trial was to account for them and all the women in his life. The passers-by, the wives, mothers, daughters of his friends. Strangers, women of the private imagination and of the imagination of the race. The nearness and farness of the female. Their everlasting hold on the reins and bridles of the imagination. Their fidelities and deceptions, fragility and persistence.
>
> All about women . . . for without women as reality, dream and idea, there would never have been such a thing as art. He admitted that.[4]

This passage demonstrates a peculiar error. Woman has been the metaphor for all that is mysterious in life, and some people have confused metaphor with its subject. As women define themselves, they will become less mysterious; while this may cripple the artist who has depended completely on the "feminine mystery," it can hardly cripple art. (Most women artists will, of course, not feel deprived of the mysterious woman metaphor at all.)

Whether by their words, tone of voice, or facial expression, many older women have communicated their interest in the subject of menopause and their almost total lack of interest in the subject of menstruation and the menstrual taboo. Some consider it an error to

* Several anthropologists have told me that when they did their fieldwork, it never occurred to them to gather data about menstruation and menopause. And in the field generally, there is little information available. What does exist is primarily concerned with menstruation, not menopause. Because of this unconscious bias on the part of anthropologists, it was necessary to make use of material—illustrative as well as textual—that was gathered by those few individuals who did research in this area, regardless of when the work was done.

combine these subjects in one book and, I expect, may take issue with the amount of attention given to the menstrual taboo.

It is obvious that menopause has a physiological connection to the menstrual cycle (there can be no ending without a beginning—the mechanisms which underlie the former also control the latter). But it has been far less obvious that the ways in which we think about menopause and even the manner in which it is experienced are, emotionally and socially, legacies of the taboo of menstruation. The image of what menopause might be, the anxiety or even horror with which it may be anticipated, are placed upon a woman from the moment she begins to menstruate.

The changes in bodily tissue, hormone levels, symptom development, and treatment of problems which are associated with menopause are discussed in detail later in this book. However, it is not possible to give full consideration to menopause if one is confined to a description of the above-mentioned events. Menopause is not a discrete event independent of the hundreds of menstrual cycles that precede it and the societal attitudes that shape woman's concept of self. It may comfort some and irritate others, but menopause occurs within the framework of the menstrual taboo and cannot be fully understood in isolation from it.

The law now codifies a woman's right to choose whether or not she will retain a conceptus. In this sense, woman has recaptured the right to control the extent to which her potential fertility is realized. The shattering of the menstrual and menopausal taboo will provide woman with respect for her body; living within the taboo, woman is trapped in a body that betrays her and defiles her.

If we don't break the taboo, we will still be ashamed of being women no matter how proud we are of particular accomplishments. Should we continue to bury the feelings of shame and pretend they don't exist, whatever self-respect we earn will be the superficial coating to a self-loathing interior. As long as we are ashamed of our bodies and the feelings which derive from their functions, we may unconsciously seek accomplishment to make up for our "fundamental uncleanliness" or unacceptability.

The pleasure of development, the acceptance of one's self, along with the accomplishments that follow from these feelings, will be only partially available to women who possess the common-knowledge opinion of menstruation and menopause.

Far beyond the natural divergence of sexual anatomy, menstruating and menopausal women differ from men in substantial ways. Why should we excise the influence of our ovaries? They do not define us per se, but they do affect the shape of female identity. The presence of ovaries and the female sex hormones is central to woman's development. Once this development is well under way we can physically do without ovaries. However, to deny their influence is to disfigure the nature of female being. To deny the ovaries is, at least in part, to turn away from our sex.

The Amazon doesn't seem to have ovaries. And she is always appealing because she doesn't need to bother with ambivalence, changes, blood, or flushes. Like the hero, she doesn't have earthly limitation. But she is merely another image of *fantasized* superiority. When we judge ourselves in comparison with her, we are always the lesser, powerless, fatally flawed. As long as women continue to believe that being female is not good enough, the Amazon will be the symbolic figure who represents escape to a better world.

The distortion of woman's image begins at menarche; it grows stronger and becomes more convoluted as long as she menstruates and experiences menopause. The distortion derives from what men think women are—and this has kept us from sharing our experiences. Menstruation and menopause do not have to continue to be secrets.

2

The Menstrual Cycle from Menarche through Menopause

In the seventh month of fetal life the ovaries contain almost a million egg cells. From then on the number of ova decreases.* At birth, the ovaries of the newborn girl contain a half-million egg cells; at puberty, ten or twelve years later, the number has dropped to 75,000. By the time a woman is fifty (give or take a couple of years), there are no egg cells left alive.†

Girl children are born with all the basic equipment and materials for reproduction. In fact, on rare occasions they menstruate shortly after birth. Infantile menstruation demonstrates the completeness of the reproductive system, but it is not an example of precocious sexual development. During the late stages of pregnancy the mother's high level of sex hormones may travel in the fetal blood supply. The newborn girl excretes these over-abundant hormones—staining is the sign of hormone withdrawal. Once these sex hormones have left, the infant's reproductive system remains quiescent until puberty.

During puberty the sex hormones, in minute supply since birth, begin active production. For boy children this means the start of sperm-cell manufacture; nighttime emissions indicate that the neces-

---

* The only other cells which constantly decrease without replenishment are those of the brain.
† The constant decrease in egg cells is no threat to the perpetuation of the species; even if 3 cells were released during every menstrual cycle between menarche and menopause, only 16,000 would have been used. Until menopause occurs, there are always far more egg cells than can ever be used for reproduction of our species.

sary materials for reproduction have developed. Girls already possess the necessary material for reproduction. Menarche, the first menstruation, is the signal that the female reproductive system is now prepared to send out egg cells from the ovaries.

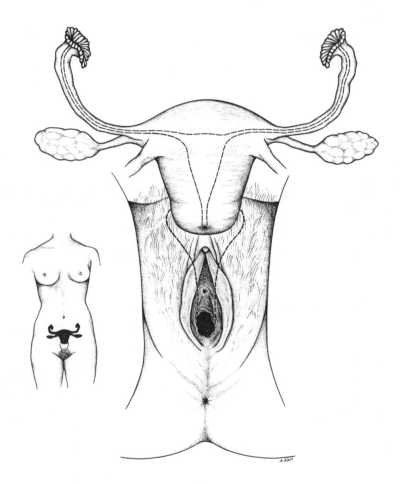

Female sexual and reproductive organs

The sex hormones control reproductive functions and have an effect on sexuality (the specific effects of these hormones on female sexuality are discussed in chapter 5). The primary organs of reproduction and sexuality, identical in the male, are separate in the female; the clitoris, after all, has no known reproductive function. This is, of course, only one of the many differences between male and female reproductive systems.

Sex hormones which begin active production during puberty have characteristically different modes for the male and female. In the male system, the sex hormones take a linear course. During adolescence the male hormones seem virtually to flood the system and then begin to taper off. After adolescence these male hormones reach a lower plateau, a level which is maintained until middle age. During middle age, the male sex hormone supply declines gradually and steadily. The most obvious behavioral effects of this linear pattern are seen in sexual activity. The interval between ejaculation and subsequent erection is shortest during adolescence and longest after middle age.

The course followed in the production of female sex hormones is cyclical rather than linear. The cycles of reproduction are about one month long. From the first menstruation during puberty to the last one during menopause, each cycle is formed by the gradual build-up of sex hormones, which peak in the interval when an egg leaves the ovaries. After ovulation, sex hormone production begins to taper off and reaches its lowest point just as menstruation begins.

These cycles are repeated four or five hundred times in each woman's life. The amount of sex hormone present in each phase of the cycle varies from one individual to the next and from one cycle to another, but the overall pattern of build-up, peak, and diminution is constant.

During puberty and again during menopause there is a discreet change in the levels of sex hormone circulating in the female bloodstream. The pubertal change reflects the switch over from low to high hormonal levels, while the menopausal change is the result of a switch from the high levels of the fertile years to lower (premenstruation) levels.

Physical, emotional, and even behavioral changes can be tied to the cyclic pattern of sex hormone activity and to the discreet changes of hormone supply between one cycle of life and the next. We know much less than we would like about the ways in which sex hormones affect women, but we know still less about the ways in which male hormones influence male feeling or action. Enough *is* known, however, to say that the pattern of hormone production is different for males and females and that this contributes to sexual differences in physical and emotional experience, as well as differences in behavior.*

* The social evaluation of these sex differences is of critical, perhaps decisive importance. As long as male experience is the guide to what is proper and

Men, after all, experience no cyclic alterations comparable to the menstrual cycle, and there is no physiological male menopause. From this point on, our concern is only with the unique nature of the female cycles of menstruation and menopause.

Puberty

The necessary plumbing is present from birth, and yet the reproductive cycles do not begin, on the average, until a girl is between twelve and thirteen years old. What starts the process of pubertal change and initiates the cycles of menstruation? This question has puzzled people for centuries. Whenever someone found a correlation between onset of puberty and any other factor, factor X was advanced as the cause.

Climate, height, weight, diet, genes, emotions, cultural advantage, even exposure to music,* have all been advanced as possible initiators of puberty and menstruation. It was suggested that the brain contains a biological clock which keeps track of the time between birth and puberty: when the hour is right, the process begins. But, as the eminent student of adolescent development J. M. Tanner queried, who or what is *reading* the clock?[1]

CRITICAL WEIGHT

In the early 1970s Dr. Rose E. Frisch demonstrated that the acquisition of a critical weight triggers the onset of menstrual cycles.[2] As we grow older, progressively more of our body composition is taken up by fat tissue in proportion to lean. During the adolescent growth spurt (one of the main indications of puberty), a girl's body composition shows a ratio of lean to fat tissue of 5:1. At menarche,

---

acceptable, female difference will be seen as inferiority. This is the current belief in our culture, and the female experiences of menstrual and menopausal cycles consequently suffer the weight of negative assessment.

* Dr. R. E. Frisch reported in *The Lancet* (May 5, 1973, p. 10007) that in the late nineteenth century an orchestra was brought to the Paris Zoo and instructed to play sweet music for the young elephants. It was later observed that elephants reached sexual maturity at an age appreciably younger than their relatives in the wild. At the time it was suggested that music had stimulated their "precocious" hormonal development.

this ratio has become 3:1.* Fat tissue has increased by 125 percent in a period of only two or three years!

The critical weight (reflecting the critical body composition) at the average age of menarche (between the twelfth and thirteenth birthday) falls between 94 and 103 pounds. At this time of life 24 percent of the girl's body composition is made of fat. Among girls who have an early menarche (nine- and ten-year-olds), and those who are later than the average (fifteen- and sixteen-year-olds), fat tissue makes up 22 percent of the body composition.

Menarche is the first menstrual cycle, but the next one or two years are a time of especial menstrual irregularity. Most of the cycles occur without ovulation during this phase. By the time most cycles include ovulation, 28 percent of the body composition consists of fat tissue. (The average weight of girls at this time is 121 pounds.)

Dr. Frisch has suggested that there is an adaptive advantage to critical weight and body composition being preconditions for menstruation. She states that in previously well-nourished women, pregnancy consumes 50,000 calories, while among those whose diet has been less rich, 80,000 calories are consumed by pregnancy. Lactation uses up about 1,000 calories per day. When 28 percent of the body composition is made of fat (and this is the point at which regular ovulation occurs), there are 99,000 calories stored. For a previously poorly fed woman, this calorie store is enough to provide *all* the energy needed to carry a fetus to term and to breast feed for one month even if the environment during her pregnancy offers scant nurture. By the time the female is able to conceive, her body has stored the necessary calories to maintain the life of the product of conception.

A critical weight, representing a critical body composition, is the trigger for menarche. Still unanswered is the question of exactly how the amount of fat tissue affects the step-up in sex hormone production. Dr. Frisch suggests that metabolic changes occurring during the dramatic increase in fat between the start of puberty and the onset of menstruation signal the hypothalamus to begin the chain of actions leading to the menstrual cycle. Whether or not this theory is confirmed, it is widely believed that the hypothalamus is the site from which menstrual cycles are triggered and controlled.

* Dr. Frisch wryly comments that the experiment at the Paris Zoo was "successful" not because sweet music induces an earlier age of puberty, but because zoo elephants eat better and exercise less than their relatives in the wild. In the zoo, they gain the critical amount of body fat much sooner.

The Menstrual Cycle

The hypothalamus is a walnut-sized collection of highly specialized brain cells, which forms the control center for several basic bodily systems (fruits and nuts continue to be the most popular sources of analogy in the anatomical world). One of the hypothalamic nuclei or aggregations of specialized-function cells controls the production of female sex hormones.*

Once the critical weight has been reached and the hypothalamus has received a message to that effect, it sends a chemical message to the pituitary gland. This gland, which is located below the hypothalamus, responds to the chemical message by producing two hormones of fundamental importance: the Follicle Stimulating Hormone (FSH), and small amounts of Luteinizing Hormone (LH)†. (Later in the menstrual cycle, the production of FSH is slowed to a halt and the production of LH increased.) As soon as the hypothalamus signals the pituitary to begin manufacture of FSH, the hormone feedback system—connecting the hypothalamus, pituitary, and ovary—is well under way; it will continue to orchestrate each subsequent cycle from the first menstruation to the last.

Three important sets of physiological events overlap in each cycle: the feedback system itself; the process of ovulation in the ovaries; and the series of cyclic changes in the reproductive and sexual organs resulting from variation in hormone levels.

---

* Other nuclei in the hypothalamus mediate responses of hunger and satiety, thirst, sexual response (at least in some species), and also play a part in emotional responses such as pleasure. The means by which the hypothalamus influences or controls these behaviors is still a subject of basic research investigation. Its role in the complex area of human behavior is by no means clearly understood. These cell nuclei are adjacent to one another, leading to the speculation that what is going on in one cell influences what is going on in others. However, it is a prodigious leap from this speculation to a lucid explanation of the workings of the hypothalamus.

Recently, a gynecologist speaking seriously offered me the following explanation of the emotional aspects of menstruation and menopause: "Emotions control the menstrual cycle and menopause. Just look at the hypothalamus." He might have said, with equal scientific justification, that the moon controls menstruation and menopause.

† FSH and LH are gonadotropic hormones. The gonads are the sex glands (in the female these are the ovaries; in the male, testes) and the target organs for the gonadotropic hormones. The gonads take up and use these hormones as they pass through the bloodstream.

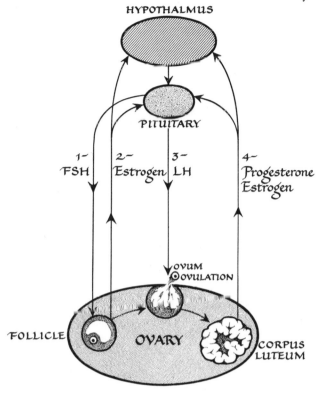

HYPOTHALMUS

PITUITARY

1~ FSH 2~ Estrogen 3~ LH 4~ Progesterone Estrogen

OVUM
OVULATION

FOLLICLE   OVARY   CORPUS LUTEUM

The hormone feedback system during the menstrual cycle. The ovulatory cycle forms the base of the diagram.

THE HORMONE FEEDBACK SYSTEM

Once the pituitary begins to manufacture Follicle Stimulating Hormone, this is secreted into the bloodstream and arrives at the ovary. (In general, only one ovary is stimulated in a cycle.) With surprising simplicity, the name of this hormone describes its function in plain English—FSH stimulates the growth and development of follicles. Each follicle contains an egg cell, and many follicles are stimulated in a given cycle. As they develop, they manufacture another sex hormone—estrogen.*

Estrogen manufactured by the ovarian follicles is secreted, and, traveling through the blood, is taken up by the pituitary gland. When

---

* *Estrogen* is derived from the Latin *"oestrus,"* which means frenzy. The principal estrogen manufactured by the ovaries is Estradiol-17 beta. Esterone and estriol are manufactured by the ovaries as part of the chemical chain which leads to production of Estradiol-17 beta.

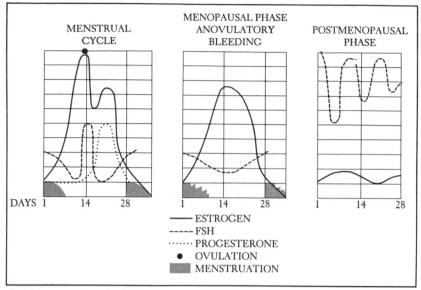

Sex hormone levels during the menstruating, menopausal, and postmenopausal years

there is a critical level of estrogen, the pituitary slows down the production of FSH and begins to produce LH. (In effect, the estrogen reaching the pituitary blocks the production of FSH.)

The feedback system continues as Luteinizing Hormone* is secreted by the pituitary gland. This hormone arrives at the ovary and changes the pattern of follicle stimulation. In combination with estrogen, LH suppresses the growth of all the follicles stimulated during this cycle—except one. This one follicle is stimulated to its full maturity, then releases the egg which it contains.†

At this point the egg leaves the ovary but the follicle remains. Once the egg is gone, the empty follicle changes its structure as a result of the action of LH to become the *corpus luteum* (yellow body). The *corpus luteum* then manufactures and secretes the second ovarian hormone of the menstrual cycle—progesterone.** (The *corpus luteum* also continues to manufacture the estrogen begun by the

---

* *Luteinizing* comes from the Latin *"luteus,"* meaning "yellow."

† When LH first reaches the ovary it causes a drop in the amount of estrogen produced. This happens because all but one of the estrogen-producing follicles of this cycle are cut off from nurture and begin to die. As they do so, estrogen supply diminishes. However, the follicle that is stimulated to mature development soon takes over estrogen manufacture with an output close to that which occurred earlier in the cycle.

** *Progesterone* is derived from the Latin words meaning "in support of gestation."

follicles in the earlier phase of the menstrual cycle.) Progesterone production keeps increasing until a critical level is reached. When this level is detected by the pituitary, it responds by shutting down the manufacture of LH. As LH production declines, the *corpus luteum* loses its source of nurture and begins to die. When the *corpus luteum* decays, the manufacture of progesterone (and estrogen) naturally decreases. (If conception had occurred in this cycle, the *corpus luteum* would have continued to flourish and the progesterone it produced would sustain fetal development until the placenta was able to take over.)

When estrogen and progesterone production reach their lowest points, another critical moment in the hormone cycle takes place: menstruation begins. During the first day or two of flow, the hormone system is relatively quiet. Then the pituitary begins to respond to the absence of estrogen by manufacturing and sending out FSH. The first stage of the next menstrual cycle, therefore, has begun while menstrual blood is still flowing.

THE OVARY AND THE EGG

The time between the manufacture of FSH and its cutoff (following the ovarian production of estrogen) is called the *follicular phase* of the cycle.* The length of the follicular phase varies from month to month and from one individual to another. However, once LH production stimulates ovulation, the *luteal phase* of the cycle has begun; its duration is more or less fixed at fourteen days. In a forty-day menstrual cycle, for example, the follicular phase lasts for twenty-six days, and the luteal for fourteen. Ovulation would occur on Day 26, *not* on mid-cycle Day 20.

The follicle which is "chosen" to reach maturity moves toward a section of the ovarian wall, again as the result of stimulation by LH. As the follicle moves, that section of the wall thins and bubbles out. In response to the surge of LH which then occurs, the follicle ruptures and the bubble in the ovary's wall bursts. The egg floats out of the follicle in fluid which the follicle contains, to pass through the

---

* It is common to speak of the first or second half of the menstrual cycle rather than the follicular and luteal stages. However, the cycle, except when it is twenty-eight days, does not break down into equal periods before and after ovulation. The luteal phase is always fourteen days, and the length of the follicular phase is determined by whatever number of days are *left* when fourteen is subtracted from the length of the completed cycle. By referring to the phases and not "halves," the asymmetrical timing of ovulation within the cycle will, it is hoped, become more widely acknowledged.

newly made opening in the wall. This is *ovulation*. Scar tissue will form over the opening (see illustration of the ovulatory cycle, page 23).

Each branch of the Fallopian tubes is attached to the uterus at its lower end; the upper section of the tube is adjacent to, but separate from, each ovary. The fingerlike ends of the tube (fribula) move toward the opening of the ovary to catch the egg as it comes through.

The egg is moved along the Fallopian tube by the hairlike cells that line the Fallopian walls and also by the peristaltic contractions of the walls. Four days pass during which the egg travels the length of the tube. During the first or second days of this journey, the egg remains viable and conception may occur, if it is joined with a sperm cell.* Should conception occur, the hormonal cycle now shifts its mode.

When fertilization does not take place, the egg begins to decay and completes its journey into the uterus where it rests upon the lining of the uterine wall. Whatever remains of the egg cell is washed out of the uterus during the process of menstruation.

CYCLIC CHANGES IN THE SEXUAL AND REPRODUCTIVE ORGANS

The uterus, which is the size of a pear, is made of muscle lined with spongy tissue, and these two layers are connected by a dense network of capillaries. The spongy lining is called the *endometrium*. It proliferates during each cycle in response to the estrogen which has reached the uterus through the bloodstream.

During the luteal phase of the cycle, progesterone combines with estrogen to stimulate even greater growth of the endometrium, and the capillaries become engorged with blood. This process of proliferation and engorgement keeps building until the ovarian hormones reach their low point, when the capillaries burst. Blood rushes out of the uterus, carrying with it most of the endometrial tissue and what is left of the decayed egg cell.

As this blood enters the vagina, it picks up some of the mucus produced in the cervix; and as it travels through the vagina, it collects dead cells from the vaginal walls. In this sense, at least, menstruation can be considered a cleansing process.

Shortly after flow has stopped, enough estrogen has been secreted by the ovarian follicles to begin the rebuilding of endometrial tissue.

---

* Sperm can reach the Fallopian tubes within a half-hour after ejaculation. Sperm cells remain viable (capable of producing a conceptus upon union with an egg cell) for at least twenty-four hours and perhaps as long as forty-eight hours after they reach the Fallopian tubes. Sperm enter the cervix within a minute after ejaculation and can stay mobile in the vagina for as long as ten hours, providing no spermicidal preparations are present.

If conception were to occur in the next cycle, the endometrium would not be expelled but would become the placenta.

Cervix

. The cervix is that part of the uterus which descends into the vagina. An opening in the cervix connects the interior uterus with the vaginal canal. It is through this opening, of course, that menstrual fluid descends and sperm cells ascend.

The cervix contains mucous glands which respond to cyclic changes of estrogen level. As estrogen increases at the start of a new cycle, alkaline and viscous mucus is produced. The thickness of the mucus covers the cervical canal, and while it does not form an airtight cap, it does serve to keep harmful bacteria from reaching the uterus. The viscosity and denseness of the mucus also lowers the mobility of sperm cells, making their journey upstream more difficult.

When LH production begins, there is a dramatic change in the quality of the cervical mucus. It becomes even more alkaline, thin, and watery.* These alterations create an optimal environment for sperm survival and transport. The creation of this favorable environment occurs *at the same time* that the ovarian wall opens and the egg cell travels into the Fallopian tube. Mucous changes, stimulated by estrogen, make entry of sperm from the vagina through the uterus and into the tubes easiest just at the time when ovulation takes place. The sex hormones work together to maximize the chances for conception.

Following ovulation, there is a dip in estrogen production and the beginning of progesterone production. Now the cervical mucus returns to its former thickness and its less alkaline makeup.

Breasts

In the luteal phase of the cycle, the breasts may become larger and more sensitive because of the combined stimulation of estrogen and progesterone. This may result in a greater responsiveness to sexual stimulation or it may make the breasts so sensitive that they become painful. As soon as the hormones reach their low point, the breasts lose this sensitivity.

* If mucous samples are taken from the cervix just before ovulation, when estrogen is at its maximum, the dried mucus takes on a fern-shaped pattern. (If ovulation occurs, the *corpus luteum* will manufacture progesterone and the luteal phase will occur.) During the luteal phase, the mucus loses its fernlike patterning. The fern test, then, done before and after the anticipated time of ovulation, will distinguish those cycles in which ovulation has taken place from those in which it hasn't.

Clitoris and vagina

The outermost section of the vaginal walls (the mucosal layer) is stimulated by estrogen and produces acidic secretions. This environment stimulates the growth of bacteria which *protect* the vagina from harmful infection-causing bacteria. The more estrogen produced, the more acid the vaginal secretion. Therefore, the vaginal environment is most acidic just before ovulation when estrogen supply is at its highest; when estrogen is at its lowest point, the vaginal environment is least acidic.*

In the luteal phase of the cycle, many women have a tendency to retain fluids and, therefore, feel bloated. Fluids are retained by many tissues, but seem to settle in greatest amounts around the uterus, vagina, and clitoris.

Masters and Johnson[3] have mapped the stages of sexual response that lead to orgasm and have observed that prior to orgasm, the clitoris and vagina become engorged with blood. The swelling during the luteal phase of the menstrual cycle exerts pressure on these organs, which may mimic the pressures of engorgement experienced just before orgasm. For some women, then, the luteal phase is a period of enhanced sexual sensation and feelings of sexual arousal.

These pressures on the vagina and clitoris continue to increase during the luteal phase. The closer to the time of menstruation, the greater the feelings of sexual arousal. For some women, however, the pressure becomes so intense that the sensation of pleasure changes to pain. With the onset of menstrual flow, when estrogen is at its lowest point, the swelling disappears and along with it the enhanced sensitivity of the vagina and clitoris.

The pacing of hormone production varies. For certain women the first day of menstrual flow, as well as the first few days after flow has stopped, may be times when estrogen production is especially low. Some women, for example, experience vaginal dryness in the first or second day after flow stops. Apparently in that cycle, estrogen supplies have not yet reached a point where they stimulate production of vaginal lubrication, and external sources of lubrication must be used to prevent painful intercourse.

* The acidity caused by vaginal secretions is not hospitable to sperm. However, the profuse and alkaline cervical mucus produced at the time of ovulation covers the sperm and protects it from this acidity. The relative loss of acidity in the vagina when estrogen is at a low level may explain why some chronic sufferers from vaginitis have their attacks just before or after menstrual flow and why estrogen loss during menopause is accompanied with vaginitis for many women.

Each menstrual cycle is controlled by the hormone feedback system. Some of the hormonal effects on organs occur in every cycle (the production of estrogen, for example, and its effect on vaginal sweating); while other changes may or may not be experienced. Of course, some cyclic responses to the sex hormones may not occur for years and then suddenly appear. Many women report that breast sensitivity isn't experienced during the luteal phase until their late twenties.

Menopausal variation

Cyclicity and the changes it stimulates continue from menarche until menopause. With menopause another discreet change begins. After twelve *consecutive* months without flow, menopause has occurred.* (This happens, on the average, at fifty years of age.) The follicles stimulated by FSH during menstrual cycles slow down and eventually begin to decay. As they deteriorate, they manufacture some estrogen but not enough to produce the critical level needed to trigger the next phase of hormone production. The pituitary continues to send out more and more FSH. Because the pituitary does not begin to manufacture LH, the luteal phase of the cycle never occurs and progesterone is not manufactured.

The follicles decay with age, but the egg cells they house immediately degenerate. Therefore, even if external supplies of estrogen were introduced, ovulation would never again occur because there are simply no more egg cells. Menopause is the end of fertility.

Estrogen is being manufactured at lower levels than in the menstruating years, but progesterone is not manufactured at all. Presumably there are other sources of estrogen supply after menopause since this hormone has been found in the bloodstream of women who have had their ovaries removed. No one, however, knows what this source is. Progesterone is also found in the bloodstream of postmenopausal women, and it is suspected that its source is the adrenal glands (located above the kidneys).

The reproductive and sexual organs are influenced by estrogen circulating in the blood and are naturally also influenced by the lowering of estrogen levels brought with menopause. One can generalize and say that the response of each organ during menopause

---

* If menopause occurs before age forty, it is labeled premature (premature menopause occurs in about 8% of women). Flow can be completely suppressed in the premenopausal years by a variety of factors which will be discussed in the next chapter. This condition is called *secondary amenorrhea*. It does not represent the death of egg cells in the ovaries, and in most cases fertility can be restored.

depends on the amount of estrogen which is lost, as well as on the *rate* at which its production declines. Rate of estrogen decline, in fact, is as crucial to menopausal responses as the absolute amount of hormonal decrease. The absence of progesterone appears to play no important role in the development of menopausal symptoms.

At menopause, when estrogen supply diminishes, each of the reproduction and sexual organs may undergo changes which are the reverse of those seen during the high-estrogen points of the menstrual cycles. However, as long as moderate amounts of estrogen are secreted, the organs show some of the same responses seen during the menstrual cycle.

When estrogen decline is severe, the uterus and breasts may shrink, the vagina will lose its sweating response, and the vaginal walls will become thinner.

What Is Normal?

Variation is the first law of menstrual and menopausal function, but *some* aspects of the cycles are fixed. For example, if menstruation occurs there must always be a high level of estrogen followed by its withdrawal. Decay of egg cells is always a part of menopause. Once the basic preconditions are realized, the experience of individual women shows enormous variability.

You can see menstrual blood or see that it is no longer occurring; but there are many aspects of the cyclic state which are not visible. With so much going on inside, and with so little known about what is actually happening, there are too many occasions for worry. Some women become anxious because menopause seems to be taking years and years. (For example, several years of erratic flow, then six months with no flow, then another year of erratic flow, etc.) Or what if one's menstrual cycles do not conform to the twenty-eight-day magic number? Does this mean that some serious malfunction is taking place, or is the reproductive cycle functioning in its normal variable way?

My periods have always been irregular and scanty. I sort of worried about this as a teenager, and had a vague feeling there was something wrong with me. I wasn't "normal." . . . The doctors never found anything wrong. . . . It wasn't until after I had a child that an M.D. was patient or caring enough to ask me what I thought was wrong. At 30, after 17 years of menstruation, I finally could believe that I was okay. This was a great joy and relief and made a lot of difference to me in psychologically accepting myself as a woman—but 17 years is a long time to worry! (K.N.D.)

For a very long time I was worried that I was abnormal because my periods were very irregular and often differed in amount of flow, premenstrual signs, etc. I had always been fed the belief that "normal" menstruation occurred for 5 days in 28-day cycles. . . . I was always terrified that I had some horrible disease but was too afraid to ask because I knew I was the only one in the world with this problem.

(A.C.)

I would like to believe that the depression and asexual feeling . . . described to me could be avoided. I would like to believe that I can experience [menopause] without displeasure or dismay. (K.P.S.)

Erratic cycles are normal during puberty and again just before menopause. And during the years in between, there is a good deal of variation, too. From menarche until the age of twenty-five, women experience the greatest amount of variation in the length of time between the onset of successive cycles.

CYCLE LENGTH

"Twenty-eight" seems to be a magic number. It has a staying power beyond rational explanation, with the result that most women seem convinced that menstrual cycles ought to be twenty-eight days in length. (Cycle duration is counted from the first day of flow to the first day of subsequent flow.) The number 28 is the result of a statistical averaging procedure in which the cycle lengths of thousands of women are added together and then divided by the number of women counted. If, for example, half the women polled had fifteen-day cycles and the others had cycles of forty-one days, the average would be twenty-eight, but none of the women, in fact, had a twenty-eight-day cycle. Of course, women do experience cycles which are twenty-eight days long, but no one has such cycles every month.

The only time when cycle duration appears to approximate the twenty-eight-day rhythm is the few years in which a woman passes her late thirties. The other thirty-odd years of menstruation are filled with cycles of great variability. It is *normal* to have cycles as short as twenty days and as long as forty-five, with every kind of variation between these points. Even if your cycle is twenty days one month and forty-three days the next, it is normal. You might worry about pregnancy during this variation, but you don't also need to worry about your state of menstrual health. As Dr. S. Leon Israel says: ". . . The absolutely regular cycle is so rare as to be either a myth or a medical curiosity."[4]

In one study, by Chiazze et al.,[5] more than 2,000 women were asked to give their cycle lengths. Fewer than 13 percent had cycles which varied in length by less than six days; 87 percent of these women had cycles which varied in length by seven days or more—counting from their shortest cycle to the longest.

The results of this study suggest that after the age of twenty-five the length between cycles becomes more stable (even though there is still irregularity). This relative stability continues through the late thirties. During the late thirties the time between one cycle and the next is more uniform than at any other time of life; cycles are still not absolutely regular, but they generally occur in intervals of from twenty-six to thirty days. When a woman reaches her forties, cycles become more variable once again.

This study had records from more than 30,000 cycles of 2,300 women of all ages. Ninety-five percent of the cycle lengths were between fifteen and forty-five days. An investigation of this scope provides much more information about cycle length than the previous reports made by individual gynecologists, which were based on their experience in practice. It has provided a more informative definition of the normal range of cycle duration than we had before. When a similar investigation is made with 100,000 women using menstrual records kept over a period of ten years, the question of normal range will be fully answered.

But Chiazze and his colleagues should be commended (and funded) for doing important research in an under-researched area. Each woman contributed an average of one year's menstrual history. This sample shows what is commonly experienced by women in one specific age group; it fails to show how the menstrual experience of cycle length varies within a woman's experience as she goes through life. Can a woman who had had a wildly varying cycle in her twenties expect to have uniform cycles in her late thirties?

Israel in his classic text on menstruation states that "Bleeding periods of from 3 to 7 days duration fall within physiological limits."*

---

* Israel bases his judgment of normal duration of flow from observations of women he saw in his practice as a gynecologist. Again, studies on much larger groups of women are needed before definition of the normal range of menstrual or menopausal experience can be complete.

Shorter or longer flow might be a sign of some abnormality; in such cases you should consult a physician.

AMOUNT OF FLOW

What is the norm for the amount of blood during menstruation? First of all, menstrual flow is real blood. The average amount of blood which leaves the uterus during menstruation is about 2 ounces in each cycle, and the normal *range* of blood loss is anywhere from 1 to 6 ounces. This is normal and *does not* lead to anemia.

Little or no research has been done on the variation in blood loss as a function of age. To do this research, blood would have to be collected and measured in each cycle over a long period of time. In the absence of research that can answer this question, we are left with anecdotal information. The experience of even a few women, however, can indicate the areas in which more research should be done and can help other women to at least begin to measure their own experience in a context larger than themselves.

As my older friends passed their thirtieth birthdays, they dropped hints of what I had to look forward to. On this list was the fact that an unnamed but very definite hormonal "upheaval" was in my future. I forgot their predictions for the first years of my thirties and only now realize that, after thirty, my cycles became shorter than they had ever been before, and my premenstrual symptoms were blessedly reduced.

Several women in their late thirties and early forties have mentioned that flow becomes much heavier for one day of the cycle. It is almost as though all the flow were concentrated in that day, and the rest of menstruation is scanty.

My friends are all in their late thirties and early forties. We would like to alleviate the ultra heavy flow that develops in these years, but we don't believe in birth control pills. (C.G.)

Heavy bleeding at this age is apparently normal. It may be annoying but it is not pathological. (The possible causes and cures of bleeding irregularities are discussed in the next chapter.)

Menstrual blood differs from other blood in our bodies in only one essential respect—it does not clot. Clots that are in menstrual discharge are said to result from the collection of blood around cervical mucus after it has left the uterus and enters the vagina.

The modifications in menstrual cycles and the variety of changes which may come with menopause are vague; nonetheless, there is a discernible pattern. Again, what is normal at one stage is not necessarily normal at another. The erratic onset, normal during adolescence and just before menopause, is not considered normal for a thirty-year-old.

Because so much of the process of menstruation and menopause is hidden (physically, culturally, and psychologically), changes in bleeding patterns of any sort often trigger anxiety. We long for a nonexistent regularity. Many of us, however, would be appalled at the prospect of having our times of flow occur in unison or finding ourselves at menopause at the same time as all our friends.

MENSTRUAL SYNCHRONY

The creation myth of the Navaho describes the life of Changing Woman. She is the single most important figure in the myth of the formation of the world of the Earth People. "Changing Woman first menstruated in the last quarter of the moon. They had Blessingway sung for her and made a blessing so all the people would have many babies. Now all women have it . . . during that time. If they don't have it then, it comes along during the full moon."[6]

In 1971, Martha McClintock published a study on menstrual synchrony among college women.[7] Studying the patterns of menstrual onset among women living in dormitories, she found that roommates and close friends came to have cycles which began on or near the same date. This synchrony, however, did not apply to women whose only commonality was sharing the same dormitory. A pattern of synchrony was also found when she studied menstrual patterns among women who work together: "The distribution of onsets [menstruation] of seven female lifeguards was scattered at the beginning of the summer, but after three months spent together the onset of all seven cycles fell within a four-day period."[8]

Whatever the cause of menstrual synchrony, it is obviously not a matter of faith or pathology. Again, this is a question which needs further study and expansion. Whatever influences synchrony, after all, influences *any* menstrual cycle. What is it that occurs on a job, for example, which influences cyclicity more than the hours working women spend leading separate lives? What effect does friendship, the sharing of a job or of a living place have on the time of onset of menopause? Is there menopausal synchrony and if so, what creates it?

There has been very little investigation into how a shared environment affects the experiences of menstruation and menopause.

Fertility Control

CONCEPTION

If a woman and her partner have intercourse on Wednesday and the woman ovulates on Thursday, she can conceive. If they don't have intercourse on Wednesday or Thursday but on Friday, she may conceive. A recently published study[9] provides data which are most startling. If a couple has intercourse any time up to and including the eighth day *before* ovulation and the third day *after*, conception may result. In the hypothetical Thursday ovulation discussed above, this would mean that intercourse without proper contraception on the Wednesday of the preceding week might result in pregnancy, as might intercourse on the following Saturday.*

It has been generally accepted that the egg cell is capable of fertilization for up to two days after ovulation, and that sperm having reached the Fallopian tubes remain viable for from one to three days. These facts led to a reproductive arithmetic in which conception was possible within a five-day period around ovulation. Indeed, this remains the most probable time of conception. The newly revised arithmetic of reproduction, however, shows that the interval in which pregnancy may follow insemination stretches from the eighth day before to the third day after ovulation—inclusive.

There are a variety of ways by which a woman might become aware of ovulation. Some women experience pain when they ovulate. (This is called *Mittelschmerz*.) Other women may have a day or two of staining at the time of ovulation, which is the result of the very high levels of estrogen circulating at this time. (This is called *breakthrough bleeding* and is perfectly normal.) More than 25 percent of women experience a discernible rise in basal body temperature right after ovulation; women can't feel or see the signs of ovulation before it has occurred. There is no absolutely reliable guide to the "safe" period because whatever the method of determining ovulation, it is always

---

* This study suggests that male births are more likely to result when the interval between natural insemination and ovulation is greatest, and that female births are more likely to follow insemination on the day before, the day after, or the day of ovulation. The inverse is true following artificial insemination, leading to the speculation that vaginal environment plays an important role in the process of sex ratio determination—at ovulation the vaginal environment may favor transport of sperm cells bearing the X chromosome.

done *after* the fact. Any contraceptive or protective measures used during the three or four days following ovulation will not protect a woman for the days *before*, and what happened on those days can result in conception. If, and only if, ovulation occurs but once in a given menstrual cycle, the safe period would begin on the fourth day after ovulation and continue until the end of the period of menstrual bleeding.

There is also no way of knowing whether or not you will ovulate more than once in a given cycle. If you use contraception only around the time you ovulated, what will happen if you ovulate again a week later with no signs? (This assumes that you didn't conceive during the first ovulatory period.) Multiple births are, after all, the living evidence of more than one egg extruded during one cycle.

To some readers this may seem like a tortured and belabored recitation of the obvious facts of life. But the facts of life do not seem to be part of our shared knowledge or even of our common sense. For example, 48 percent of those answering the menstrual survey said that conception is most likely to occur during mid-cycle, 20 percent answered that ovulation was the time when conception was most likely to occur; those who believed that conception would most likely occur fourteen days before menstruation could be counted on the fingers of one hand. Among those who said "mid-cycle" were those who had good reason to doubt their own veracity:

*It's supposed to be the middle of a cycle, but I never could understand how I had a full term baby, nine months to the day from when I married, when I'd finished a period two days before the 4th (Sept. 4 to June 4).** (L.J.N.)

After six unplanned pregnancies using the rhythm method, I can only believe there is no "safe" time for me. (C.C.)

I understand the "normal" time for conception is midway between periods. However, I became pregnant five days before my next period should have begun.† (R.L.C.)

The conviction that the cycle is twenty-eight days long is probably responsible for a good part of this confusion. If cycles were predictably twenty-eight days in length, then ovulation *would* occur at mid-cycle—fourteen days after menstruation and fourteen days before the next.

---

* Had L.J.N. not become pregnant she would have found that her next date of flow was about twenty-one days after her last period.
† Again, had R.L.C. not become pregnant, she would have found that her flow came about eight days later than she anticipated.

Almost 80 percent of women who used Planned Parenthood facilities in 1973 took oral contraceptives. Thirty-five percent of the women who answered the menstrual questionnaire used the pill. While the pill completely suppresses ovulation and therefore offers 100 percent protection from pregnancy, it may contribute to the confusions concerning the time of ovulation and the most likely time for conception.

The forgetfulness of women taking oral contraceptives is understandable—there are enough things to worry about without keeping track of the time of ovulation when ovulation isn't even occurring. However, if and when a woman goes off the pill (and women are doing just that in increasing numbers), she will find herself back in a world where ovulation and conception regularly occur and she won't have the vaguest idea when. Whenever women change methods of contraception, counseling about conception should definitely be given.

CONTRACEPTION

The Pill

There is no perfect method of birth control. This statement will come as no surprise to most women but might puzzle many physicians who feel they have the answer in pill form.

Oral contraceptives contain synthetic forms of estrogen and progesterone. These externally supplied hormones assume some of the functions of the internally manufactured ovarian hormones and block others. Synthetic estrogen and progesterone build up the uterine lining and also suppress ovulation, but once the pill is withdrawn, the endometrium breaks down and menstrual flow occurs. When the pills are resumed, the lining is rebuilt.

The pill, of course, is not perfect because its side effects range from the mildly annoying (nausea) to the potentially fatal (thromboembolism).

The pill seemed to be a perfect method until its side effects were widely publicized. It not only offered 100 percent protection from pregnancy but could also regulate menstrual cycles for the millions of women troubled with erratic times of onset and relieve menstrual cramping as well. Among the 35 percent of the women answering the menstrual survey, 97 percent reported one more change after taking the pill, and in most cases they felt the change was for the better:*

* Among those reporting positive changes, 23% said flow was lighter and they had less cramping, while another 42% said flow was lighter.

My flow is less heavy and lasts for five not seven days. It is also more regular. (B.K.)

Much less pain and cramping, about 75 percent less flow. (B.B.P.)

Makes it last for 2–6 hours—lovely. (L.M.S.)

My flow is lighter and my "premenstrual tension" is more intense. (R.H.T.)

Yes, the pill does regulate flow but, as Seaman points out, it can also end it altogether: "It is no longer just a vague worry but an established fact that a certain number of women simply do not start having their periods again after they stop taking the pill. Others have irregular or scanty periods. In either case, they may find that they cannot conceive. They are sterile."[10]

There is some evidence that the women most likely to have menstruation suppressed altogether are those who were irregular before taking the pill. In other words, the very women whose physicians recommended the pill because it would bring menstrual irregularity under control may find themselves never again having to worry about menstruation *or* fertility.

Whatever a woman's feelings about menstruation or fertility, her decision to use birth control pills is based on the knowledge that they are an effective contraceptive—she is not volunteering for sterilization or menstrual suppression. There may be women who would choose to take the pill even if they were told there was a chance that fertility and/or menstruation would be permanently ended, but every woman has the right to make an informed choice. There is no question but that good medical practice includes a discussion between a physician and his patient about this potential "side effect" of oral contraceptives before the woman makes her choice of method.

When I took the pill my period was reduced to nothing. I went through all the physical feelings of getting my period, but no flow. (M.R.)

M.R. went off the pill and her cycles returned. This does not always happen. And no woman should have to undergo the anxiety and anguish of waiting to see if menstruation (and fertility) will come back.

While almost all observers of pill side effects state that cramping and heavy flow are reduced, premenstrual tension and irritability may increase:

I was on the pill for three years—it lessened my flow, but I was "bitchy"
all the time. (M.O.K.)

Many physicians recommend the pill for women who suffer from
menstrual pain. While the pill does cure cramping in many cases, it is
not a universal panacea. Several women, for example, reported that
when they told their doctors that menstrual cramps had returned
despite use of the pill, their physicians said, "Well, if *that's* the case,
the pain must be in your mind!"

IUD's

For a few years in the late sixties and early seventies, IUD's were
also subjected to "miracle method" promotion. Loops, coils, springs,
or T's that are made of copper or plastic, IUD's are mechanical
devices inserted into the uterus. Exactly how they prevent conception
is not known. Some suggest that the presence of foreign material in
the uterus creates a higher white cell count—and it is the white cells
that kill sperm. Others suggest that the presence of foreign material
causes the uterus to contract much more than it does normally, with
the result that the conceptus cannot lodge itself in the endometrium.

For many women, the use of IUD's results in much heavier menstrual flow and increasing cramps. Among 13 percent of the women
who answered the questionnaire and who use the IUD, 73 percent
have reported these side effects:

Cramps are the bulk of my menstrual problem. . . . I never had
severe cramps until my IUD was inserted. My gynecologist prescribed
some painkillers, but they leave me too woozy to function. (J.L.W.)

I never, never had any cramps or other feelings of the "curse" until I
had an IUD inserted. . . . (V.D.C.)

However, even with contraception, there are those women with
different menstrual reactions:

For some reason when I got my IUD I stopped having cramps. (D.E.S.)

At first it increased my menstrual flow tremendously the first two days
of my periods, but shortened the length of the period. Now, after four
years, it seems to have just shortened my period. (K.S.)

At first, IUD's were said to offer 99 percent protection from pregnancy. That number has now dropped to between 96 and 98 percent
protection. In 1974, the Dalkon shield (inserted in the uterus of one
out of every three users of IUD's) was implicated in the deaths of

several women and was taken off the market for six months. When it was reinstated we were told that the device would be safe if it were inserted properly. Because improper insertion may be apparent only when trouble (either minor or life-threatening) develops, women may not find this reassurance very comforting.

Diaphragm

The diaphragm is used in conjunction with a sperm-killing cream or jelly. It is put in the vagina before intercourse and serves as a mechanical barrier preventing sperm from entering the opening of the cervix. It also functions as a stable container for spermicide, keeping the cream or jelly securely placed over the cervix during intercourse.

Diaphragms and spermicides have *no effect* on the hormonal cycle nor on the organs of sexuality and reproduction. They do, however, have one menstrually related effect: with a diaphragm in place during menstruation, intercourse does not result in blood-stained sheets. This will be of special interest to the nineteen women who said they refrained from intercourse during menstruation because of messy sheets. In fact, women who use other methods of contraception might consider getting a diaphragm just so it can be used during menstruation.

The diaphragm, which offers 97–98 percent protection from pregnancy (when used correctly and regularly), has no harmful medical side effects and may even protect women from V.D. and vaginal infections, was, paradoxically, not declared a miracle—in fact, it almost passed into complete obscurity. In 1961, just after the pill came on the market, 74 percent of women using Planned Parenthood selected the diaphragm; but in 1973, only 4 percent were asking for diaphragms. By 1974, however, interest in the diaphragm was restimulated as disappointment increased with the "perfect," newer methods.

Breast feeding

Some women believe that while they nurse they cannot get pregnant again because nursing inhibits ovulation. However, this is not always true—nursing does not necessarily inhibit ovulation.

After the birth of a child, the sex hormones go through a period of rearrangement. They readjust from the very high levels produced during pregnancy to the lower levels needed for menstrual cycles. (The same kind of readjustment occurs after an abortion or miscarriage.) The time required to complete the period of readjustment is not fixed, and there is no way of predicting when the feedback system controlling menstruation will be back in operation. Because ovulation may well occur before the reappearance of menstruation (this would happen, for example, if the first cycle after a pregnancy were ovulatory), conception could occur without your ever being aware that you were fertile. Instead of seeing menstrual flow, you would go for a pregnancy test.

Another factor plays an important role in the resumption of menstruation during nursing. Critical weight represents the amount of stored calories necessary for the completion of pregnancy plus a month of lactation. Because breast feeding burns 1,000 calories per day, a woman who has had a poor diet and has a low amount of fat stored will take longer to reach the critical weight (and resumption of menstruation) than a woman who has had a rich diet.

Breast feeding *cannot* be relied upon as a method of contraception. The pill should not be used during nursing and opinion varies about the time when an IUD may be safely inserted following pregnancy. During the time you are nursing, use a diaphragm or foam-plus-condom.

Menopause
The average age at which menopause occurs in our society is fifty years. It can occur prematurely (as early as one's thirties), and it always follows surgical removal of the ovaries. Within this age range, twelve or more *consecutive* months without menstruation indicates that menopause has been completed. Then and only then can you throw away your birth control devices and not be concerned about pregnancy. (Of course, surgical removal of the uterus even if the ovaries are intact also ends fertility.)

Before menopause there are erratic cycles for as much as two or three years. You may not menstruate for months, only to begin once again. Don't assume that menopause has been completed and fertility has ended before twelve consecutive months.

And others . . .
Condoms, foam, condoms-plus-foam, cervical caps, and rhythm are methods of contraception which are less reliable than the pill, IUD, and diaphragm. Condoms-plus-foam and the cap seem to offer greater protection than condoms alone or rhythm, and can be used if more effective methods are not available or cannot be used.

A good deal of attention has been given to the shortcomings of gynecologists (and still more attention would be profitable), but little to the ways in which women carry the responsibility for controlling fertility. The use of any of the three most reliable methods (pill, IUD, and diaphragm) means that women have the entire responsibility for birth control. It isn't news that women have not always demonstrated an unfailing sense of responsibility in this area.

For a short time I worked in an abortion clinic. One day I was counseling a woman who had come in for an abortion. I began to discuss the possible methods of contraception she could use in the future (she had been using rhythm), and I asked her what method she planned to use after the abortion.

"Rhythm," she answered. "I used it for eleven months and it worked!"

At the proven rate of success for her chosen method of contraception, she would be back at the clinic once a year.

Thus far I have had one child conceived two days after a period and once conceived while a prophylactic was used. I have therefore recently added the diaphragm as a last defense against unwanted pregnancy.

(R.F.)

"Why" I ask, "is the diaphragm the *last* defense?" This is the first time this woman will have chosen a reliable method. Presumably she could have acquired a diaphragm earlier on.

Actually I haven't used it [the diaphragm] yet and since I have had sex, I experience anxiety over whether my period will occur or not. When I took the pill I never worried. I stopped the pill because of concern for my health and am not totally confident of the reliability of the diaphragm and so hesitate to use it. (J.N.)

Until a method of controlling fertility that is 100 percent effective and 100 percent free from harmful side effects has been developed, women will have to use the available birth control methods wisely and faithfully.*

Whatever the method of contraception, the decision should be based on what you think is best for you. Honest self-appraisal is as

---

* Male-controlled contraceptive methods may be perfected in the future. I should think, however, that before large numbers of women will trust men with the responsibility for birth control, men must more fully demonstrate their responsibility for the results of conception. We will need to see a man's concept of virility separated from his need to impregnate regardless of the feelings of his partner.

important to the success of a contraceptive as is honest information about its effects and side effects.*

If you choose the pill, know its side effects before starting. You now know that it is perfectly normal to have shortened duration of flow, or less flow, as well as more regular cycles. (It is *not* normal to have no flow at all. If flow stops, go off the pill, but get another method of birth control right away.) If you select an IUD, you know that heavier flow and cramping are not peculiar responses to the device, but perfectly normal (although not perfectly acceptable) side effects to its use.

"Normal" can mean free from pathology or it can mean the statistically arrived-at average. When a woman is concerned about her menstrual cycle or about the changes of menopause, information about what is normal rather than pathological is, obviously, both a guide and a reassurance. However, the knowledge that a menstrual or menopausal experience is statistically normal can lead to a double bind. Because so many other women suffer the same problems, we think we shall not complain; yet the problem is difficult to live with, and it doesn't go away just because we have plenty of company. The "normal" experiences may not be at all acceptable.

* *The Birth Control Handbook*, published in Canada, and *Our Bodies, Our Selves* both give thorough reports on the various contraceptives, their correct use, and their side effects. *The Birth Control Handbook* may be ordered by mail from P.O. Box 1000, Station G, Montreal, Quebec H2W2N1.

3

"Complaints," Causes and Cures

Menstruation and menopause are the only physiological processes in which mild to severe discomfort is a normal accompaniment to healthy functioning. Fifty to 75 percent of menstruating women suffer some degree of premenstrual syndrome (PMS) distress, and 85 to 90 percent suffer one or more symptoms of menopausal syndrome (MS).* These syndromes are not manifestations of disease, but are the by-products of normal functions of the reproductive system.†

The description of normal menstrual and menopause processes enables us to appreciate the elegance and delicacy of the hormone system and the interplay of hypothalamus, pituitary, and ovaries, but the existence of PMS and MS leads to the observation that nature's design can also be astoundingly crude.

Physiological malfunction and disease can occur within each of the body's systems; the reproductive cycle is no exception. Pathology, however, is always an exception to ongoing bodily function. The widespread incidence of difficulty associated with the normal (non-pathological) function of these cycles demands special attention. Are the menopausal and premenstrual syndromes, truly, examples of

---

* Seventy-five to 80% of menopausal women suffer one or more symptom, another 10% suffer severely and are at least partially incapacitated.
† In itself, the magnitude of this is shocking. Even more shocking, however, is the failure of the scientific and medical communities to address themselves to the causes and cures. Suggestions for the means to change this situation are given in chapter 10.

nature's imperfection or are they the result, rather, of environmental stresses?

Because these syndromes are found among every social and economic class, any environmental stress which is to be their cause must be all-pervasive. Some MD's have said that the tensions of modern-day life offer an adequate explanation of cause and prevalence of the menstrual and menopausal syndromes. But Scully points out: ". . . The evidence is that Indian women had considerable difficulty with their monthly periods. Over all the Rocky Mountain region, numerous herb remedies were used to induce normal menstrual flow."[1] And after reviewing evidence from twenty-four cultures around the world, Janiger *et al.*, concluded:

> This study does not . . . substantiate the opinion that the predilection for symptoms of menstrual distress follows the degree of comfort and complexity of living. It seems consistent, however, with the thesis that premenstrual distress is a universal phenomenon and is subject to great individual variation in the incidence, nature and severity of its symptoms. These do not seem to follow any consistent cultural pattern . . . and do not seem to favor any particular etiological hypothesis.[2]

Excesses of physical duress and hardship are not to blame for the widespread incidence of menopausal or premenstrual syndromes. What about the effects of societal stress? Again, this stress would need to be of a sort that reaches every class and would have to be found throughout history.

Menstruation has been judged a negative part of life for thousands of years in virtually every case where information is available. (This social history is reviewed in chapter 4 and further analyzed in chapter 6.) The societal meaning attached to menopause varies from one culture to another. In our culture it has negative connotations. It is not possible to separate the experience of either menstruation or menopause from the social evaluation placed upon either occurrence, if we consider the difference that the social context makes in the evaluations of feelings.

Childbearing in our society is considered a wondrous event—as long as a woman doesn't exceed the agreed-upon quota. Many women tend to have good feelings about the emotional and physical changes going on during pregnancy. Assuming that a woman wants the child she is carrying, its kicks and turns are sources of pleasure rather than pain. Even if she does feel discomfort or pain, these are "positive" feelings because pregnancy is culturally a positive condition.

Now imagine a woman with menopausal flushes. Society places no priority on the experience of the older woman. In fact, in our culture there is little if any place for her at all. At best menopause is considered somewhat ludicrous, and at worst it is labeled a disqualifying crippler. Negative social attitudes are so pervasive that only the most extraordinary woman can consider a flush pleasurable rather than discomforting.

The need to have some fresh air during the flushes will be perceived by most people as still another pathetic problem of menopause; women will try to hide such a condition to avoid ridicule or discrimination. The myriad idiosyncrasies of pregnancy are benignly smiled upon because they are "charming," and the needs of pregnant women are usually met with speed and indulgence. (The one who assists often feels as if a service is being proffered to the species.) The pregnant woman is given every reason to feel pride, while the menopausal or menstruating woman is given every reason to feel shame.

Societal evaluations and responses are not the primary cause of the physical changes of pregnancy, childbirth, menstruation, or menopause, but they certainly affect the ways in which women experience these changes. Pain and discomfort are not imaginary sensations: the extremely high levels of sex hormones produced during a pregnancy tend to create a sense of physical and emotional well-being; the low levels of these hormones just before menstruation and during the menopause may create physical or emotional distress. However, the intensity of each sensation is increased or lessened by the context in which it is experienced. There is no way to predict successfully just how women's feelings during menstruation and menopause will change when the cultural taboo is dissolved. Some of the problems will remain the same, others may change, and still others may disappear completely. But the overall experience will be very different, and the tensions that have come from the taboo will, let us hope, disappear.

What are the premenstrual and menopausal syndromes? What can be done to alleviate the unacceptable, though statistically normal, byproducts of menstruation and menopause? What are the abnormalities of menstruation and menopause, and what can be done to cure *them*?

Premenstrual tension is a relatively common condition, which in common with . . . "menopausal misery" causes a great deal of suffering in patients and yet has received scant attention by the medical profession. . . . There are probably three main reasons for this: the first is that they are benign subjective conditions, so that no obvious harm will come to the patients even if untreated; the second is that women have come to accept these symptoms as inevitable ills; and the third is that the majority of the profession are male, and, never having suffered personally from these complaints, do not take them seriously.[3]

Premenstrual Syndrome

In the late 1930s, Dr. R. T. Frank created an umbrella term, *premenstrual tension*, to describe those problems associated with the normal experience of menstruation. Some twenty years later, Dr. Katharina Dalton, working with women suffering from menstrual difficulties, began to use the term *premenstrual syndrome* to cover a multitude of problems:

> Characteristically, patients with premenstrual syndrome have more than one symptom. Apart from tension, sufferers from premenstrual migraine [for example] may also complain of premenstrual bloatedness of the abdomen, breast tenderness, and spells of giddiness. The presence of multiple symptoms leads to patients being wrongly classed "neurotic," as formerly were many sufferers from other endocrine disorders like diabetes, myxedema or Addison's disease, before biochemical investigations led to a positive diagnosis.[4]

Ninety percent of the women who answered the menstrual survey reported one or more premenstrual symptom. Of these, 24 percent had symptoms which were physical and included weight gain, constipation, diarrhea, backache, and headache. Eighteen percent of the respondents experienced problems which might be classified as emotional—including depression, irritability, insomnia, and unprovoked crying; 46 percent reported premenstrual symptoms which were both physical and psychological. Only fifty-seven women, 10 percent of the total responding, said they had no premenstrual symptomology. In some cases an individual woman is not aware of a particular pattern to her feeling—but others are:

> It is estimated that from 25 to 100 per cent of women suffer from some form of premenstrual or menstrual emotional disturbance. . . . Eichner makes the discerning point that the few women who do not admit to premenstrual tension are basically unaware of it, but one needs only to talk to their husbands, or co-workers to confirm its existence.[5]

It is sometimes difficult to recognize the presence of the premenstrual syndrome because its symptoms can be found at any other time of the month. In fact, a symptom becomes associated with the syndrome only when it recurs with some regularity just *before* or *during* the time of menstrual flow.

A syndrome . . . multiple causes . . . how can you tell if you've got it? For some women, of course, this question would be answered by a forced smile and clenched teeth. These people have no doubt about it, they know all too well that each month there are a series of changes—many of which are not very pleasant. For other women, however, only a minor change or two may be observed, and still others have no idea that anything at all is happening that is related to menstruation.

Dalton recommends that women keep a menstrual calendar. Give yourself enough space to note down the days when you are menstruating and a letter code for the symptoms you experience any day of any cycle. You can underscore letters when symptoms are severe or you can use capital letters for this purpose. After several months you can look back over your calendar and see what pattern, if any, is formed. If a given symptom or several symptoms always cluster around the time of flow, *you* have the premenstrual syndrome.

When I first kept a menstrual calendar, I became depressed noting the times I felt bad. Instead of keeping separate records, I made a code for good feelings as well as bad and recorded it in my appointment book. These are some of the observations made by women who didn't need a special chart in order to identify symptoms:

Approximately one week prior, I bloat up, feel fat and klutzy, get very irritable, cramps, back and leg aches during. (J.M.)

No real distress except melancholy which I actually enjoy. It's a quiet reflective time for me. (R.J.C.)

My skin breaks out around both ovulation and my period. My temper is short; I am near tears, I am depressed. One fantastic thing—I have just discovered that I write poetry just before my period is due. I feel very creative at that time. (K.A.M.)

Best time emotionally and physically begins during menstruation. At midpoint I feel a downward shift. Most tense time is just prior to my period when physical and emotional states are at their worst. Symptoms vary from month to month. (F.G.)

I become a cross bitch about 4–7 days before my period, snap at my

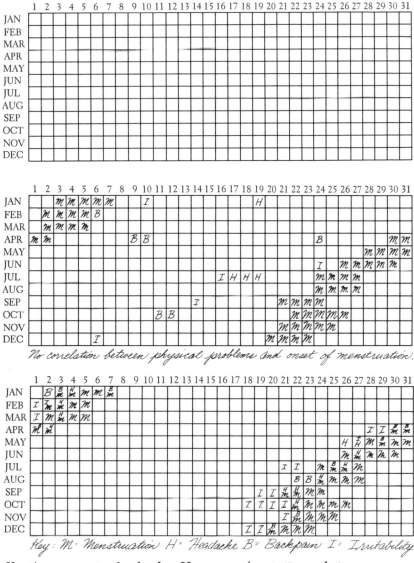

No correlation between physical problems and onset of menstruation.

Key: M: Menstruation H: Headache B: Backpain I: Irritability

Keeping a menstrual calendar. Here are a few patterns that may emerge
when recording physical and emotional states during many consecutive
cycles. The markings on the third calendar suggest the presence of the
premenstrual syndrome.

children for nothing, put down my husband, can't stand loud noise,
get shaky if I have to deal with stress. My period's arrival brings me to
a more optimistic frame of mind. Then, immediately after my period
it's as if I have shed something emotionally, for then I feel ready to
take on some new projects, lose a couple of pounds and set new goals

for myself! About midway between periods I can almost determine the moment of ovulation by a changed taste in my mouth. I now begin to crave sweet snacks until my period arrives. Naturally unusual events can obscure this pattern somewhat. (K.C.)

I am as witchy as hell just before the flow starts. (B.B.W.)

About a week before, my breasts seem to swell and they hurt like hell. Almost exactly seven days before I get a severe migraine which lasts a day—sometimes I throw up. . . . The symptoms haven't characterized the entire twenty-two-year span of my periods. They've occurred separately and together. The migraines were characteristic of my late teens and twenties. (ANON)

A few days before my flow is to start I feel the need for extra sleep at night, and if I don't get it I become easily irritable. Also more often than not, I get a "cleaning urge" and will clean the house, etc., with unending energy. The day I start I feel a relief and am glad the whole process is continuing okay. (N.C.H.)

Clearly, not every "symptom" of the premenstrual syndrome is discomforting. Some women enjoy the changes they experience each month.* In some cases of premenstrual syndrome, two aspirin every four hours will be a complete cure. But what if the migraine you thought only came at random intervals, or depression or insomnia, is always associated with the time of menstrual onset? Learning to identify a symptom as part of the syndrome leads to greater understanding of the problem, but it certainly doesn't tell you what can be done once this condition is accurately identified.

TREATMENTS

There is no universally agreed-upon treatment for premenstrual syndrome because little attention has been paid to the causes of the problem. Those who have studied PMS are faced with a difficult problem because so many symptoms are found:

> We are merely beginning in our scientific understanding of premenstrual tension. Perhaps one reason has been the use of a single variable or single etiology approach. Clearly a . . . multilevel approach is necessary to understand this complex interaction between hormonal shifts, early learning and development, conscious and unconscious conflict and cultural reinforcements.[6]

* Naturally, not every woman is going to find melancholy a positive experience. Still, because of the overwhelming negativity directed toward menstruation (and menopause), many of us lose sight of the alternatives available when confronting a cyclic change of feeling.

Putting aside the theories based on the premise that PMS is "all in your mind" (discussed in chapter 6), and the theory of the culture as a reinforcer (discussed in chapter 4), there is still another theory of PMS—as a side effect of the physiological processes regulating the normal menstrual cycle.

Some scientists say that PMS is caused by hormone imbalance; others claim it is the result of retention of water or salt. Poor diet, lack of adequate exercise, and mineral deficiencies all have vocal proponents, and each theory suggests a particular method of "correct" treatment. In the absence of a generally agreed-upon cause for PMS (and in the presence of the confusion that results with multiple hypotheses), women are free to evaluate theories and treatments and choose the one which seems most acceptable.

Lack of exercise

Timonen and Procopé[7] suspect that inactivity may contribute to the severity of premenstrual symptoms. After studying the menstrual experience of competitive athletes and gymnasts, they found that athletics has a "strikingly favorable effect" on the premenstrual syndrome. While there was a dramatic reduction in the incidence of headache and tension associated with menstruation, premenstrual swelling, premenstrual cramps, and constipation were not reduced at all. However, *cramping during flow* was less commonly experienced among the athletes.

The researchers offer this hypothesis to explain their findings: Swelling before menstruation leads to poor physiologic brain performance. Continuous physical exercise (a fact of life for athletes) increases the circulation to the brain, and in effect, overrides the limitations caused by the swelling. They conclude: "It seems obvious that the need for physical exercise is not sufficiently satisfied in modern society. Facilities and guidance ought to be available explicitly for mass sports. Evidently mankind has strayed too far from a natural manner of living to find the way back without guidance."[8] While lack of adequate exercise may make the symptoms of PMS more severe, it is not the cause of the syndrome's initial appearance.

Hormone imbalance

Dalton is the chief proponent of the theory that premenstrual syndrome is caused by a hormone imbalance in which there is too little progesterone in relation to estrogen. This imbalance can occur in two ways: an over-abundance of estrogen may be produced in the

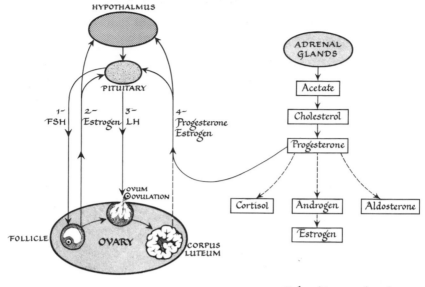

It has been suggested that where ovarian levels of progesterone are too low, the ovaries will utilize progesterone from the adrenals.

follicular (pre-ovulatory) phase of the cycle, swamping the system and blocking the functions of progesterone produced in the luteal phase. There is also the possibility that normal amounts of estrogen are produced during the follicular phase but that less than average amounts of progesterone are manufactured in the luteal phase.

Dalton believes that low production of ovarian progesterone is the primary cause of menstrually related symptoms. She comes to this conclusion in the following way. Under normal conditions, the ovaries manufacture the progesterone needed for proper reproductive function and the adrenal glands produce chemicals that are eventually transformed into a group of hormones known as the *corticosteroids*. During the process of chemical transformation, progesterone is manufactured. As the chain continues, adrenal progesterone is altered and, eventually, corticosteroids are produced. Under normal conditions, then, it has nothing to do with the sex hormone cycle of the pituitary-ovary-hypothalamus.

When the *corpus luteum* manufactures less progesterone than usual, the reproductive system appropriates progesterone from the adrenal chain. The feedback system of the sex hormones is then able to continue and the menstrual cycle is completed.

Despite a lack of ovarian progesterone production, the menstrual cycle remains unbroken, but this occurs at the *expense* of corticosteroid production in the adrenal glands. The chain leading to the production of corticosteroids is broken when progesterone is removed from the adrenal glands, and, as a result, fewer corticosteroids are manufactured. A little hormone snatching leads to a large number of unpleasant repercussions.

> The adrenal glands produce many corticosteroids, each with a different function. Some are responsible for the water balance in the tissues of the body, others regulate the sodium and potassium in the cells, some prevent allergic reactions, others regulate the level of the blood sugar and some mobilize mechanisms responsible for protection of the body from bacterial and viral infections. . . . The progesterone [of the adrenals] is the precursor, from which, after many more chemical reactions, the many and varied corticosteroids are formed.[9]

The many different kinds of symptoms in the premenstrual syndrome, according to this theory, result from the depletion of corticosteroids. This theory is certainly logical, but is it also an exposition of what occurs? One indication of its accuracy would be found if progesterone were administered to women who suffer from premenstrual syndrome. If too little progesterone were the cause of the symptoms, then added amounts of progesterone would alleviate the symptoms.

Dalton has been treating women who have premenstrual syndrome for more than twenty years. She reports that when pure progesterone is used, the remission of symptoms is complete in nearly 100 percent of the cases.[10] Synthetic progesterone (properly called *progestin*) may be successful in treatment, as may some estrogens which are broken down into progesterone in the body. In her opinion, however, pure progesterone is the only certain successful medication. The synthetics are worth trying first because they are less expensive.

Having suffered with premenstrual syndrome, I read Dalton's reports with special interest. With such a high rate of success, I wondered why a gynecologist had never suggested it as treatment for PMS in all the years I had been asking for relief. I interviewed several prominent New York City gynecologists and each stated that he had tried progesterone therapy in the treatment of PMS. In most cases they found that it did not dramatically relieve these symptoms. These men were not familiar with Dalton's work. While they did occasionally treat patients with progesterone, if the problem still persisted after one treatment they would abandon it instead of varying the dose and trying to find the proper amount for an individual. In her findings, Dr. Dalton has underscored the need for individualized dosage, noting how the responses of the patients who received the same amount of progesterone varied markedly.

I then spoke with Dr. Herbert Kupperman, a well-known endocrinologist and strong proponent of long-term estrogen replacement therapy; I thought he might at least be open to Dalton's suggestion that progesterone replacement therapy is an effective means of controlling menstrual symptoms. In his opinion, the doses Dalton has reported successful in curing symptoms are too small to have any physiological effect. This implies, of course, that it is Dalton's belief in the cure which is successfully transmitted to her patients.

When questioned further, Dr. Kupperman reported that he did not have very much first-hand experience with the treatment of premenstrual syndrome. (This is not surprising since treatment by an endocrinologist is very expensive. Should a woman with PMS try to use clinic facilities in order to get endocrinological help, she will most likely first have to go to the gynecology clinic and she may never get past it. While such clinics seem to believe that menopausal syndrome is a hormone problem, they do not take the same view of PMS and rarely, if ever, refer PMS women to the endocrinology clinic.) I pointed out to Dr. Kupperman that since he was committed to the treatment of menopausal syndrome as a hormone deficiency condition, there might be sound logic to a similar cause for PMS, and this would demand hormonal analysis and treatment. Kupperman retorted that if every woman with premenstrual syndrome went to see an endocrinologist, the physicians would be swamped and unable to offer treatment to anyone else.

Dr. Kupperman made an informed judgment when he said he thought the amounts of progesterone used by Dalton were too small to be effective. Although he had not tested her hypothesis, he seemed content with his evaluation that mental suggestion was responsible for the cure—an assumption he would never make about estrogen treatment and menopausal syndrome. His disinterest in the problems of premenstrual syndrome and his theory of its cure (by will rather than chemicals) reflect just another way of sweeping PMS under the rug.

Dalton could not give me the name of one physician in the United States who is currently working with progesterone as a replacement therapy for premenstrual syndrome. When we consider the millions of women who suffer from PMS, it is shocking that so little attention is paid to finding a possible cure. This is further demonstrated by the reports of women who responded to the menstrual questionnaire: among this group of 558 women, 86 percent said they had one or more premenstrual symptom. Many reported on treatments they had tried, but not one woman said she had ever been given progesterone!

The most obvious way to study the usefulness of progesterone replacement therapy would be a large-scale study using the double-blind design. Half the women would receive progesterone and half a placebo. (The study would have to engage large numbers of women in order to administer different doses to subgroups.) Neither the woman nor the person giving the medication would know who was getting what.

Some studies have been done where *progestins* (synthetic progesterones) have been compared in effect with tranquilizers, or diuretics, or placebos, indicating that progestin is not very successful in alleviating premenstrual symptoms. Although progesterone is expensive, it would have to be used in the study of premenstrual syndrome before a fair evaluation of its use could be made.

Under some circumstances, the estrogen in the body, which can be a progesterone antagonist, acts to block the effects of injected progesterone. If too much estrogen is produced, then the effects of progesterone would be stopped. Even if this is the first step leading to PMS, the results would quite possibly be the same as if progesterone were underproduced—the adrenal progesterone might still be snatched away from the adrenal chains in order to complete the menstrual cycle, and progesterone as a replacement therapy would still be necessary.

Of course, it is also possible that PMS results from hormonal abnormality when neither of the sex hormones is in abnormally high or low concentration. Many women may have a built-in sensitivity or allergy to either hormone, so that while the production of sex hormones would proceed at the usual rate, another aspect of the physical system could violently react against the hormone—or be completely unresponsive to its presence. In this case, the physical system would respond as if the actual production of sex hormones were in disarray. Gilman says: "By grading the responses of women to the same and different amounts of estradiol, it has been possible for the first time to present definite evidence for the existence in women of estrogen-sensitive and estrogen-resistant types."[11]

Whether or not estrogen (or progesterone) sensitivity or resistance is the cause of premenstrual syndrome, treatment of the syndrome with hormone replacement is made more complicated by this sensitivity or resistance. A very small amount of sex hormone may do wonders for one woman who is sensitive to the compound but nothing for the woman who has a natural resistance.

It has also been suggested that PMS results from a menstrual toxin produced the week before menstrual flow. Once menstruation occurs, the production of toxin stops (until the week before the next flow). One group of researchers claimed to have isolated this toxin but were unable to identify its chemical composition before the vial in which the isolated toxin was stored broke.

Water retention

Weight gain, swelling, and feeling bloated are among the most common symptoms of the premenstrual week. These symptoms vary in degree—as do so many other aspects of menstrual and menopausal experience. Some women gain a pound or two just before menstruating, while others may add as much as 10 to 15 pounds. This temporary weight gain is the result of water retention in the body tissue.

Some of the effects of water retention are obvious. Indeed, anyone who regularly gains 10 pounds in the premenstrual week will say the results are more than obvious and may need a second set of clothes to accommodate the change. Some of the side effects, however, are less easily seen in relation to their cause. Dalton mentions that:

> A common characteristic of women with premenstrual syndrome is that although they may be healthy, energetic and active . . . they have great difficulty in standing still for long. This inability . . . is related to water retention and a tendency for the water (and blood) to accumulate in the feet. . . . These are the school girls who faint after standing too long at morning assembly, and the women who edge themselves . . . against the walls at cocktail parties.[12]

Some physicians believe that *all* symptoms of the premenstrual syndrome can be traced to water retention. Or rather, the symptoms can be traced to salt retention because it is the salt contained in the cells that attracts and holds the water. Depression, for example, is said to result from too much fluid surrounding the brain; and irritability, another common symptom, results from the response of nerve cells to an imbalance of sodium and potassium. (One part of the transmission of messages along the nerve cells results from the exchange of sodium and potassium across the cell membrane. If there is an excess of sodium, the normal balance is disrupted and hyperirritability may result.)

There are two main methods of controlling the amount of excess fluid held during the premenstrual week. A reduction in salt intake and an avoidance of high salt foods should mean less tendency to retain fluids. If this method does not succeed, diuretics are available.

Diuretics flush excess water out of the system quite successfully; however, they also remove potassium, which is not in excessive supply. Whenever taking diuretics it is essential to replace this potassium—either by eating high-potassium food (like apricots and bananas) or by taking potassium pills.

On a practical level, the problem of water retention can be solved. On a theoretical level, there seems to be greater difficulty. Because some physicians believe that *all* symptoms of premenstrual syndrome should be removed along with excess water, what happens when only some of the symptoms disappear?

The many symptoms which may remain after water is flushed out of the system might lead theorists to conclude that water retention is not *the* underlying cause of premenstrual syndrome. Timonen and Procopé very quietly suggested this in their findings on exercise and PMS. If vigorous exercise and increased circulation alleviated some symptoms but left bloat and weight gain untouched, then it is possible that these last two symptoms are unrelated to the others. For some doctors, the conviction that water retention is the cause of all the real symptoms of premenstrual syndrome remains fixed despite contrary evidence. The theory is right but the patient is wrong. What remains after the water is removed is not part of the physical syndrome but rather the result of some imbalance in the patient's mental state!

> This concept gains support from the fact that symptomology is so often out of proportion to the quantity of salt and water retained, and that psychotherapeutic measures apparently influence the cycle in some cases. Certainly the preoccupation of the physician with metabolic minutia to the exclusion of psychologic and emotional factors is almost certain to lead to failure in treatment. To emphasize the importance of psychological factors in the genesis of clinical manifestations of this syndrome, the term "psychological edema" has been suggested.[13]

According to Thorne, if swelling isn't in the tissues it is in the mind, because swelling must be the cause of the syndrome—no matter what.

Although 70 percent (or more) of women have symptoms of the premenstrual syndrome, the number of symptoms and their intensity varies from one cycle to the next. Why does this great variation exist and why, in my case, for instance, does it seem related to the length of cycles? Why do all signs of premenstrual syndrome disappear when my cycle is twenty-five rather than twenty-nine days, and why do the symptoms seem almost crippling when the cycle shifts to thirty-two days? These questions still remain unanswered.

Menopausal Syndrome

The *climacteric syndrome* is the technical name for all the symptoms associated with the transition in sex hormone levels during a fifteen-year period. During this interval the female sex hormones change from the high levels of output during the fertile years to a new and lower baseline which will remain fairly stable for the rest of one's life. Although it is thought that the symptoms related to menopause (the cessation of menses) occur near the time of menopause, symptoms of menopausal change can and do occur at any time during the climacteric period.

Considering the statistics, it is absolutely normal to have symptoms along with the climacteric. Or rather, it is normal to have one or more symptoms as long as they don't interfere with the discharge of responsibilities or the carrying out of regular routine. Eighty percent of women passing through menopause have one or more symptoms, but only 10 percent have such severe symptoms that they interfere with daily routine. For this 10 percent, symptoms are considered abnormal. It is, of course, also abnormal from a statistical point of view to be one of the 10 percent of women who have absolutely no symptoms with menopause—but this is an abnormality no one worries about. (It would be extremely interesting and useful to learn why these women have no problems.)

In discussing the menopausal syndrome, then, we are talking about both the "normal but not acceptable" and the abnormal manifestations of hormonal change. The causes and cures apply to both cases of the menopausal syndrome.

There is no method of predicting which woman will have symptoms of menopause or how severe the symptoms will be, even with a previous history of menstrual difficulty or problems in childbearing.

Eighty to 90 percent of women experience the menopausal syndrome, but only 30 percent of menopausal women seek medical attention to relieve these symptoms. What are the symptoms which prompt women to consult their physicians and seek relief? Levine and Doherty cite:

. . . the classical "symptoms of the menopause": flushes of the head, face, neck and chest, profuse sweating, sensations of cold in the hands and feet, dizziness or faintness, headaches, irritability, depression, insomnia, pruritus (intolerable itching and tingling) of the sexual organs, constipation, and increase in weight.[14]

Other symptoms associated with menopause include menstrual flooding or scanty flow, wildly fluctuating intervals between cycles of flow, dryness and thinning of the vaginal walls, increased vaginal infection, and loss of breast firmness. More serious conditions of the post-menopause include atherosclerosis (fatty deposits in the arteries) and osteoporosis (brittleness and porosity of the bones). The symptoms (except for the last two) may appear before, during, or after menopause. When they appear before, it is generally in the two to three years before flow is completely stopped.

Hot flashes or flushes (the terms are used interchangeably) are perhaps the most famous or infamous symptoms of the menopause. Intense flashes or waves of heat suddenly sweep through the upper half of the body, often provoke a red face, profuse sweating, and sometimes are accompanied with feelings of suffocation. Each of these conditions results from rapid changes in the diameter of blood vessels.

No one knows what physiological change triggers the vascular alterations. The flushes might result from the erratic swings of estrogen and progesterone since estrogen lowers the body temperature and progesterone raises it. However, erratic swings of hormone production are characteristic of the changeover from prepuberty to the time of menarche, yet adolescent girls do not have hot flushes. It has also been suggested that they are a result of estrogen deprivation or of an abundance of Follicle Stimulating Hormone (FSH).* Others have maintained that the flushes result from the over-activity in the pituitary (over-activity coming from the continuous job of manufacturing FSH). Each hypothesis is questionable; none is true for all cases. When younger women have the physiological conditions that are said to cause flushes, flushes do not occur.

Among women of menopausal age, there are certain women who don't get flushes at all and others who may have only one or two bouts. For some women, though, flushes recur almost one on top of the next, causing severe discomfort. There is little a woman can do on her own to avoid them because they can be provoked by almost any

* When estrogen production is low, the pituitary manufactures FSH; it keeps on with this until the ovaries have produced a high level of estrogen. During and after menopause, the ovaries are no longer able to produce high levels of estrogen and the pituitary, therefore, keeps manufacturing more and more FSH, which is secreted into the bloodstream.

normal situation that changes the body temperature—this includes everything from getting under the covers to becoming emotionally upset!

Atherosclerosis is a contributing factor to heart disease, and it is not coincidental that once past menopause, atherosclerosis becomes a health problem for women. Below the age of fifty (the menopause average), twice as many men as women suffer from heart disease. During the menstruating years, women have a lower risk of heart disease—a protection lost at menopause. Once a woman is past menopause, the incidence of heart disease equalizes.

Osteoporosis affects 25 percent of women of postmenopausal age, whereas in men it is a disease of advanced age. The vertebrae may compress, causing back pain and even malformation (i.e., Dowager's Hump). Because the bones become brittle, the danger of fracture following a fall also increases.

SURGICAL MENOPAUSE

Hysterectomy is the name for the surgical procedure in which the uterus (or some part of it) is removed. The ovaries are not necessarily removed during this operation although this frequently happens.

Surgical removal of the ovaries. This operation, performed in 1809, marks the beginning of abdominal surgery.

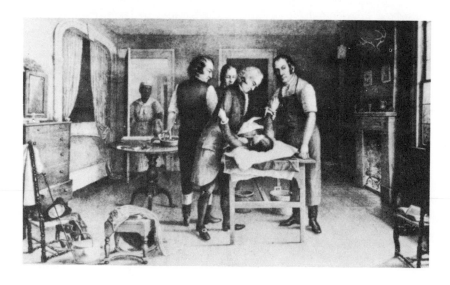

Many women, in fact, who have had hysterectomies don't know whether or not they still have ovaries.

When the ovaries (both of them) are surgically removed, menopause occurs *immediately*. The symptoms which follow ovarectomy when it is performed on older women are the symptoms of menopause, and they are usually severe because the drop-off in estrogen is not gradual as it is under most normal conditions but sharp and absolute. After the operation there are no ovaries to produce any estrogen or progesterone.

Because a severe menopause may follow after both ovaries are removed, older women should make sure to have a thoroughgoing discussion with the surgeon before he performs abdominal surgery—especially if it is to be a hysterectomy. "Adult ovarectomy has been, and sometimes still is, recklessly included in surgery for hysterectomy. Usually it is unnecessary and undesirable and should be expressly forbidden by the patient when she signs the operation permit, particularly if she is not yet postmenopausal," say Money and Ehrhardt.[15]

In the best of all possible worlds, it would be advisable to leave the decision about removing the ovaries to the surgeon, since abdominal surgery is major surgery and is a strain on both one's health and one's pocketbook. If, upon getting a look inside, the surgeon finds badly diseased ovaries that are life-threatening and you have signed a release only for the removal of your uterus (or whatever organ is the target of surgery), he will have to leave the ovaries in. Then, after you have recovered from the first operation, you will have to go through major surgery a second time to have your ovaries removed.

Because so many needless ovarectomies have been performed and because it is often impossible to find a doctor who really listens to what you want, it may be most sensible to follow the suggestion of Money and Ehrhardt and sign a release only for the previously arranged purpose of surgery. While some women will need to have a second operation, many will not and will live with intact ovaries. This group of women will be spared an unnecessarily abrupt and trying menopause.

Of course, whether menopause occurs naturally or follows surgery, not every woman gets every symptom, and in many cases the symptoms that do appear are short-lived. Symptoms like atherosclerosis and osteoporosis, however, are serious; if they could be prevented the result would be a healthier and longer life for women after menopause. What can be done to prevent or cure symptoms of the menopausal syndrome? What is the cause of the syndrome?

CAUSES

Hormone imbalance

Physicians and medical researchers generally agree that the primary cure for most and perhaps all manifestations of the menopausal syndrome is estrogen replacement therapy. "When the symptoms of the menopause are really troublesome, especially the hot flushes, there is no better, no more specific therapy than estrogen. Whether or not such treatment, once initiated, should ever be discontinued remains a matter of controversy."[16]

Because estrogen replacement therapy cures many of the problems of the menopausal syndrome, estrogen deprivation may be the source of the syndrome. In chapter 2, the role of estrogen in cyclic alteration of reproductive and sexual organs was noted: as estrogen levels increase, the uterine lining is built up, vaginal sweating and cervical mucus increase, and the vaginal environment becomes acidic. When estrogen supply diminishes, and especially if this happens over a brief period of time, each of the areas once stimulated by estrogen shows evidence of deprivation.

A lack of estrogen, then, may cause the uterus and breasts to shrink, the vagina to lose its sweating response, the cervical mucus to diminish, and the vaginal environment to become relatively more alkaline. When vaginal walls thin, the distance between the vagina and urethra becomes so small that the risk of urinary tract infection increases. The changes in vaginal environment, of course, make the risk of vaginal infection greater.

Symptoms of emotional change include depression, irritability, nervousness, and insomnia, and can be provoked by a broad spectrum of events (internal and external) or may develop in response to the presence of the physical symptoms of the menopausal syndrome. When the sex hormones are at their lowest point in the menstrual cycle, many emotional symptoms occur. Such symptoms, then, might also be expected during the interval when estrogen production is shifting to a low postmenopausal level.

Some women produce sufficient amounts of estrogen well into their seventies and never experience any sign of menopause except the loss of fertility and flow. Others have a slow and steady decline in estrogen production and experience mild symptoms which may appear for a short period of time only. When the change from the high-estrogen levels of the menstrual cycle to the low levels of the post-menopause is abrupt and of great proportion, women will probably experience severe symptoms of the menopausal syndrome.

The relationship between rate of estrogen decline and severity of symptoms is easily seen when studying the effects of surgical menopause. From the instant both ovaries are removed, menopause occurs. Removal of the ovaries, of course, causes the immediate end to fertility as well as the end to production of the ovarian sex hormones —estrogen and progesterone. The loss is absolute, and the body experiences the most drastic changes from its previous hormonal baseline to no ovarian hormones at all.

If the ovaries are removed after the menopause, the effects of hormonal loss are much less dramatic than if surgery occurs before menopause. If the ovaries are removed in women below the age of thirty (give or take a couple of years), the subsequent symptoms are not severe. This fact has led some people to question the premise that menopausal symptoms are caused by estrogen deprivation, since estrogen deprivation is as great in a surgical menopause at twenty as it is at forty.

Others have suggested that the reason for the mild symptoms following surgical menopause in young women and the severe symptoms after surgery in older women can be explained by habituation: the cells become accustomed (or addicted) to high levels of estrogen. The longer they are exposed to estrogen, the more profound the addiction. By the age of thirty-five or forty, the cells are completely habituated and the body responds to an abrupt decrease in estrogen by producing withdrawal symptoms.

The withdrawal theory would also explain why the suggested causes of hot flushes do not hold when applied to young women. The theory has a compelling logic, but only future research will reveal its soundness.

CURES

If a woman has only mild menopausal symptoms she may not seek medical attention, while she might seek relief from occasional bouts of insomnia or irritability. Tranquilizers are often prescribed. (Valium, it appears, is the world's most popular tranquilizer.)*

---

* While tranquilizers help reduce tension, aid sleep, and relieve anxiety, their abundant use reflects a medical attitude that lacks depth and responsibility. This is especially true for the long-term prescription of tranquilizers. All too

When symptoms are more severe or more troubling, estrogen replacement therapy is often prescribed.

A woman consulting a physician for relief of menopausal problems will be examined and her history taken. Part of this preliminary examination may include a vaginal smear. The smear is analyzed and rated according to the amount of estrogen present (sometimes this rating is called a *femininity index*—a misnomer of cultural importance).

The vaginal smear, of course, has nothing whatever to do with femininity nor, in fact, does it reflect the amount of estrogen circulating in the bloodstream. The vagina has a strong response to any estrogen that is present, and so a vaginal smear that shows a good response in terms of estrogen may only mean that there is no problem in the vagina! (Eighty percent of vaginal smears taken a decade after menopause show a good vaginal response to estrogen, but most certainly 80 percent of patients have low estrogen levels at this time.)

The amount of estrogen can be determined by an analysis of blood or by analyzing a twenty-four-hour output of urine. These techniques are more costly than the estrogen analysis of vaginal smears but they are much more informative. It would be most valuable if estrogen assays were taken at decade intervals starting after age thirty; the physician would then have a clear picture of the relative decrease in estrogen production. Of course, this is rarely if ever done. (In fact, it may only be part of the experience of relatives of endocrinologists and the very wealthy.)

After an analysis of estrogen output, the physician makes his assessment of the need for estrogen. Even without an analysis that shows particularly low amounts of estrogen, the physician may decide to begin estrogen replacement therapy if the symptoms are severe or troubling.

Estrogen replacement therapy (ERT)—the controversy

The controversy about estrogen replacement therapy (ERT) in the medical community does not center on the value of this therapy, on

---

often this represents an easy way out for a physician who does not want to take the time or trouble to treat the menopausal syndrome—especially in cases where diagnosis is elusive.

It is also especially important that women understand that some of the emotional responses during menopause are reactions to external situations—situations which would have to change before the emotional stress was alleviated. Blurring the feeling of tension, of course, may make living with the situation possible, but it does nothing to change it.

which there is widespread agreement, but about the timing and duration of its administration.

The argument is between those who believe treatment should be started *before* symptoms appear and should continue for the rest of a woman's life, and those who believe it should be started *after* symptoms appear and be discontinued after six months or a year and not resumed unless symptoms reappear.

Those who believe that ERT should begin before symptoms are seen, consider menopause (and not just the menopausal syndrome) a deficiency condition. They believe that the female body requires a good supply of estrogen through life and that the lack of estrogen creates a deficiency state. Treatment should be started as soon as estrogen begins to diminish (in the late thirties or early forties) and should continue for the woman's lifetime. Kupperman says:

> It may well be that the human female, because of the advances of medicine, now lives much beyond her reproductive potential. . . . She is then exposed to the exigencies of ovarian estrogen deficiency. It is for this reason that we feel that the climacteric syndrome, presenting with or without symptoms, warrants continued longterm estrogen therapy; thus one would treat the estrogenic deficient female in much the same way one would treat a thyroid deficiency—whether or not there is a presenting symptomology.* [17]

Kupperman's statement expresses the logical basis of the deficiency theory. Some of the proponents of this theory go on to make claims for ERT which are extravagant. In *Feminine Forever*—and by "feminine" he meant forever full of estrogen and young—the late Robert A. Wilson assured his reader that the saggy skin of middle age would, upon treatment with ERT, become "smooth, supple and taut again." He went on to assure us that:

> *Menopause is completely preventable.* No woman need suffer menopause or any of its symptoms if she receives preventive treatment *before* the onset of menopause.

---

* Science and medicine, of course, cannot be charged with the full responsibility for the early demise of the ovaries. Scientific advances have only made it possible for us to become aware of the discrepancy between the limits of the human life span and the limits of the ovaries.

Certainly it is sensible to have fertility end by the age of fifty; it may not be at all sensible to have the production of ovarian hormones decrease. However, in this case nature had no means of correcting an error in design—sexual selection being an obvious impossibility once fertility ends—women have had to live with the results of nature's error. Since nature cannot be self-corrective in this case, science and medicine will have to do the job. And women will have to see that it is done.

Menopause is curable. Under proper medical treatment, nearly all symptoms cease in the vast majority of cases.[18]

Not all of Wilson's assertions are misleading or overstated. Many of the symptoms of menopause will not appear if treatment with ERT is begun before symptoms develop, and many symptoms will be cured once treatment is begun. However, read carefully; he blurs at least one important distinction. Menopause, after all, will occur, with or without ERT. The ovaries will not extrude any more egg cells and so fertility will definitely end. No matter how much external estrogen is supplied, the ovaries themselves will stop producing fertile levels of estrogen and progesterone. None of the symptoms of menopause that result from estrogen deprivation, of course, will develop if estrogen is replaced before they appear.

Members of the opposing camp believe it is bad medical practice to treat women with ERT before symptoms appear. They do not consider menopause, *a priori*, a deficiency disease. Only evidence of the menopausal syndrome is an indication that treatment is in order. Treatment will be discontinued after an interval and will not be started again unless symptoms appear again. If symptoms do not appear after treatment has ended, the treatment is considered complete.

There is no way to resolve this dispute about the correct pacing of estrogen replacement therapy, but the forms of estrogen used are the same whichever approach is used.

The three most common estrogens used in ERT are *conjugated estrogens equine* (such as Premarin), *ethinyl estradiol* (also used in oral contraceptives), and *diethylstilbestrol* (DES is used in the morning-after pill).*

Ethinyl estradiol in contraceptive form has been linked to increases in blood clots and thromboembolism (stroke). The risk of stroke increases with age and, for this reason alone, it would be wise to use one of the other estrogens in replacement therapy. There are other reasons, too. Oral contraceptives often have the side effects of weight gain, tenderness of the breasts, headache, and nausea. Because these are among the symptoms one is trying to cure with ERT, it makes little sense to use ethinyl estradiol. Kupperman says:

* When purchasing prescription medicines, the generic name for the medication is almost always cheaper than the same drug ordered by its brand name—conjugated estrogens equine will cost less than Premarin, for example, and the same is true for progestin and Provera.

We prefer to use the conjugated estrogens equine, the so-called "natural" estrogens . . . because they are not associated with many abnormalities that have been noted with the synthetic steroids. . . . They are remarkably free from nausea-inducing effects, and they seldom have the adverse effects on skin pigmentation which has been seen with other estrogens. . . .

The effect of estrogen upon thromboembolic phenomena has not been seen in patients receiving the conjugated estrogens for long periods of time. The incidence of abnormal vascular changes in these patients is practically non-existent in contrast to those patients who have been observed while on contraceptive pills.[19]

Conjugated estrogens equine would appear to be safer than other forms of estrogen. A true statement of the health risk in long-term replacement therapy cannot be made until careful, controlled studies are done and until larger numbers of women are using ERT. Any woman who volunteered for such a study, like any woman who now chooses ERT, is a guinea pig and a gambler, hoping that the benefits will outweigh the risks.

The gamble may not be nearly as great as that associated with use of the contraceptive pill. During the fertile years, the ovaries produce large quantities of estrogen and the pill dumps still more estrogen into the bloodstream. During the menopausal years and those that follow, much less estrogen is produced and the hormone externally supplied is bringing estrogen back up to the normal levels of the fertile years. With ERT, the body is getting no more estrogen than was freely present for the thirty or forty years of menstruation; there is little reason to assume that unhealthy responses will occur in a healthy woman. Nonetheless, it is possible that after menopause, externally supplied estrogen might have some ill effects, and this problem must be studied.

ERT should not be started if a woman has abnormal uterine bleeding, since this may be a symptom of uterine cancer. The source of the bleeding should be diagnosed and the problem (whatever its origin) successfully treated before initiating ERT. ERT should not be used by women who have had cancer of the breast because estrogen has been linked to the growth of already existing cancer of the breast. Even if a woman believes her breast cancer is completely cured, the risk is not worth the benefits of ERT.

If ERT is an appropriate treatment for an individual woman and she chooses it, it will generally be given in cyclic form. Long-term, uninterrupted estrogen can result in breakthrough bleeding. Because of the increased rate of uterine cancer in older women (the only symptom of which may be uterine bleeding), breakthrough bleeding needs to be avoided, since there would be no way for a woman or her doctor to be sure that irregular bleeding was a result of too much estrogen or a sign of pathology.

When ERT is cycled, bleeding is *scheduled*—it follows the withdrawal of treatment in most cases. Withdrawal bleeding always occurs if estrogen is used in conjunction with progestin. The most common method of using ERT is two weeks of estrogen, followed by a week of estrogen plus progestin (often Provera), and a week of rest. During the fourth week bleeding occurs. In effect, a menstrual cycle has been re-created by the use of externally supplied sex hormones, and the endometrium is built up and shed each month. If bleeding occurs at any other time of this cycle, treatment must be terminated until the source is diagnosed and treated.

Estrogen may work wonders or it may do very little. For many women it cures most of the troubling side effects of menopause; and for some, ERT is the source of an enhanced feeling of well-being even though they were not troubled by the menopausal syndrome.

I had 10 years of menopause (starting at thirty-nine following surgery) and suffered mental distress. I wished I could go back to menstruating again. All is under control now, with my estrogen replacement therapy.

(D.M.R.)

One gynecologist said: "Medical science can't do anything more for your depression. For breast pains all I can suggest is you wear a supportive brassiere." The endocrinologist I saw prescribed estrogen which I took for six months with no results. When I reported this to him he became angry and said, "You have deep psychological problems! I suggest you see a psychiatrist." My regular doctor, a woman, who referred me to both the men, can now only suggest Valium.   (J.H.)

Periods every two weeks starting at age forty. Excessive bleeding. Great emotional distress and loss of energy due to frequency of periods. Premarin and Provera relieved symptoms.   (C.F.)

I happen to be one of the . . . women who had absolutely no symptoms at menopause except the cessation of bleeding. I was menstruating normally until age fifty-four and then stopped. After starting estrogen replacement therapy (six years later) I would meet people who had not seen me for a while and who kept on remarking how well

I looked. I did not think about it until I suddenly realized that these remarks started after I had begun ERT. . . . I have not developed Dowager's hump or the dryness of the vagina that makes intercourse painful. (R.P.)

Women who have troubling symptoms at menopause and who cannot take estrogen may be treated with androgen. Women whose only menopausal symptom is loss of sex drive may be treated successfully with androgen, which is also sometimes used to cure PMS. Androgen is a male sex hormone produced in small amounts by females. (Similarly, small amounts of estrogen are produced by males.) The dosage of androgen which is effective in treating menopausal symptoms is sufficiently large that it may produce some masculinizing changes (deepening of the voice, growth of facial and body hair, etc.). If the treatment is immediately discontinued these symptoms will disappear, but if treatment continues they may become permanent.

Estrogen replacement therapy is not the modern-day equivalent of the Fountain of Youth. However, it may prevent or cure some conditions which could shorten a woman's life. This is the case with atherosclerosis. Fatty deposits in the arteries which contribute to heart disease are rare in premenopausal women, but at menopause and after, the rate at which women suffer this condition equals that of men. There is reason to believe that ERT prevents atherosclerosis or at least reduces its incidence.

ERT can prevent some of the conditions which result in premature ageing among women. (Osteoporosis, brittleness, and porousness of bones are found in elderly men, but they occur in 25 percent of menopausal women.) ERT can prevent or cure some of the conditions which may make a quarter of a century or more of a woman's life less pleasurable. (Dryness in the vagina leading to pain during intercourse is almost always cured with the use of estrogen.) If a woman wants it, ERT is easy to come by, unless she is looking for a physician who will use estrogen as a preventive measure and begin treatment *before* any symptoms are evident. There are a number of reasons why this is true.

Conventional medical school training for the most part bypasses the subject of preventive medicine and fails to educate doctors to focus on nondisease factors (such as diet and exercise) which influence symptoms.

Unless a woman is in a menopausal "crisis," she will receive little attention when discussing menopause. Like premenstrual syndrome, menopausal syndrome does not generate a sense of drama—at least not for the physician; the conditions are experienced by perfectly healthy women and the symptoms may be slow to appear. All of this adds up to a situation in which neither medical training nor the physician's self-concept as savior is likely to help him help his patients. Besides, he is a participant in the culture that views "female complaints" as woman's fate.

If the symptoms are severe, a physician will of course do all he can to relieve them. (This is not the case with PMS, however.) But if the symptoms are relatively bearable or have not appeared, and he finds his patient in good health, he will tell her that whatever is happening is an acceptable part of a normal process. His patient may be labeled a complainer if she persistently demands relief, or she may be called a worrier if she asks for treatment before symptoms appear.

There is another very important reason why ERT as a preventive measure is not more widely practiced. In many cases, women are reluctant to embrace any long-term treatment which involves hormones. However, this "reluctance" deserves a closer look. Millions of women are using synthetic estrogen in order to prevent pregnancy, even though the estrogen used (ethinyl estradiol) may cause harmful and sometimes dangerous side effects, while conjugated estrogens equine, used in the management of menopause, appears to be free of these effects.

It may be that menopausal women are just smarter than younger women and do not want to experiment with hormones but would rather wait until further studies are done. However, there is more good reason for menopausal women to use estrogen therapy than there is for younger women to use contraceptive pills—much more. (The estrogen levels of menopausal women are much lower, and ERT is the accepted treatment for some symptoms. Fertile women can choose other contraceptives.)

The discrepancy between the vast number of younger women using oral contraceptives and the small number of women using long-term ERT may be explained in another way. Today it is generally considered to be an act of good citizenship to limit the size of families, and while the pill isn't 100 percent safe, it is 100 percent effective. More important than patriotism is the fact that the pill is the *only* form of contraception that has no direct contact with the genital or reproductive organs—it enables the user to separate sex and reproduction. If the genitals are "unclean," the pill is the cleanest form of birth control.

By considering ERT a woman is implicitly making two statements: Menopause exists, and it need not be an infirmity. She is making a positive statement about herself in the face of a negative social assessment of her value.

Estrogen replacement therapy is not the perfect solution to menopause or menopausal problems. It is not perfect because we aren't yet sure it is perfectly safe; and it is not perfect because it is neither appropriate for every woman nor a cure for every symptom. However, it is the best *medical* method available to women thus far, and it does cure or prevent a wide range of menopausally related symptoms.

One of the most essential lines of investigation for the future would be to establish the conditions (internal and external) that affect the amount and rate of estrogen decline during menopause. In what ways do eating habits, amount of exercise, vitamin intake, and amount of sleep, for example, affect the production and circulation of estrogen?

Some women have reported that Vitamin E and the B vitamins reduce many menopausal symptoms, including hot flashes. Others say that Vitamin C brings excessive flow under control. Adelle Davis states that adding calcium/magnesium supplements to the diet can prevent osteroporosis and, of course, the use of polyunsaturated fats may reduce the chance of getting atherosclerosis. Such regimes are surely worth a try because they are self-administered and relatively inexpensive, but only future research will give us a guide to their effectiveness for large numbers of women. This should be high-priority research . . . and yet it is not. If women knew the answers to these questions, we would be in a position to change our habits and so control the production of menopausal symptoms.

No one can assure women that ERT is absolutely safe or that it will cure all their menopausal problems. And some menopausal problems are responses to the society's evaluation of the older woman's status (this subject is explored in chapter 9). Until more research is done, each of us, using the information that is available, is on her own. The experience of friends, the opinions of physicians can be a guide, but you must make the choice.

Menstrual Pain

Menstrual cramps may be the symptom of an illness. A complete physical examination, including a pelvic, and thorough medical history should be done when menstrual pain is severe. After an examination you will know whether there is a pathological condition or if, instead, you are one of the millions of women who experience pain with menstruation (*dysmenorrhea*).

Most of the women who answered the menstrual survey reported some problem with menstrual cramps. Many women who say they do not have cramps often mean they don't suffer from debilitating pain. It is rare to meet a woman who has never had any menstrual cramping.

Talking with women who, like myself, have worked as counselors in abortion clinics, I found that it is the rare woman who looks puzzled when her counselor remarks that the procedure will feel like menstrual cramps. I only met one client who said she'd never experienced such a thing.

When menstrual pain is severe it may be accompanied with vomiting, nausea, and/or diarrhea. Until the past few years, dysmenorrhea was widely considered more a figment of women's imagination than a fact of menstrual life. Fortunately, this distorted assessment has begun to lose popularity, although many gynecologists still maintain such views. (A brief historical survey of attitudes toward menstrual pain is given in chapter 6.)

As long as doctors and their patients believed that pain was a reflection of neurosis and therefore not "real," women lived with misery—either not seeking relief or not finding it.

Having been plagued by dysmenorrhea for thirty-two years and having seen several physicians about this, I can truthfully say that they would offer very little help, excepting the various medications like "Darvon," etc., that did not relieve the pains. I even tried acupuncture once. It helped during the pains but not as a preventive measure. Most physicians do not feel that menstrual cramps are "serious"—they treat the whole thing offhandedly. I can assure you that I am looking forward to menopause. (R.P.)

All the years I was menstruating, I was always a little uneasy about my cramps, thinking maybe it was all in my head, maybe I was making it difficult for myself because I did not really think menstruation was all that great a boon. In spite of calculated efforts to brainwash women into thinking like this, I am convinced that it was not psychological, psychosomatic, or whatever.

When our baby was born, we made a frantic trip to town (35 miles) and the nurse commented that I must have had some pretty strong

*labor pains because she could feel the baby's head already. My reply
was that I didn't know, I'd never had a baby before, but that I'd had
menstrual cramps lots worse than the labor pains I'd been having. . . .
The nurses and the doctor roared with laughter at my wonderful sense
of humor. I wasn't joking—I had had cramps worse than that all
my life.* (A.M.H.)

Menstrual cramps are real pain and very little is known about either
their cause or cure. This isn't surprising since the problem has only
recently become a "legitimate" medical issue.

Dysmenorrhea is most widespread among women between the ages
of fourteen and twenty-five. (During the first year or two after menarche, cramps are relatively uncommon.) When women with a history of dysmenorrhea take oral contraceptives the problem usually
goes away, although some women report that after being on the pill
for a year or so the cramps come back.

Most cycles in the year or two after menarche occur without ovulation, and ovulation is completely suppressed by oral contraceptives.
These facts, combined with the observations above, have led some
scientists to conclude that dysmenorrhea only occurs in cycles in
which there hasn't been ovulation. This theory, however, does not tell
us why dysmenorrhea lessens after the age of twenty-five, why women
on the pill sometimes have cramps, and why dysmenorrhea stops after
some but not all pregnancies.

In an article called "Evaluating Dysmenorrhea," M. J. Daly has
suggested that menstrual pain is the result of uterine oversensitivity
to progesterone. Normally the uterus is always contracting but we
don't feel it. According to Daly, the uterus can have an overly
sensitive (almost allergic) response to progesterone produced during
the cycles and will contract much more than normal. These intense
contractions lead to pain. He goes on to speculate that this sensitivity
is likely to be greatest when progesterone is first introduced into the
system—the years after menarche; as the uterus becomes used to its
presence, the sensitivity declines. Similarly, during a pregnancy the
body is flooded with huge amounts of progesterone which may effectively lead to a desensitization of the uterus. Daly's hypothesis does
not account for the pain felt by older women or the pain felt by
women who have given birth to children.

Dalton believes there are two types of menstrual pain: *spasmodic
dysmenorrhea*—the name for cramping that starts on the first day of
flow and comes and goes in sharply felt waves; and *congestive
dysmenorrhea*, which is felt as a dull, aching pain that often begins

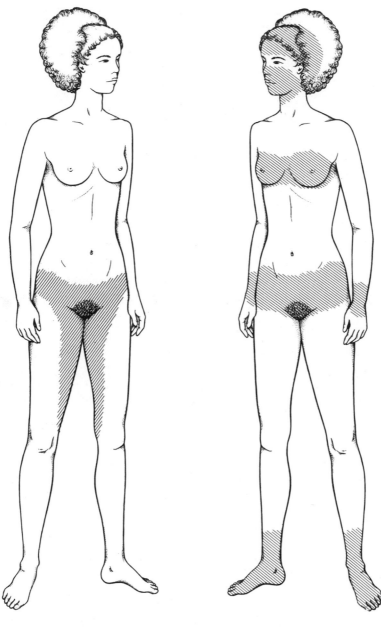

SPASMODIC
DYSMENORRHEA

CONGESTIVE
DYSMENORRHEA

Two types of menstrual pain. The gray area at left is site of discomfort in cases of spasmodic dysmenorrhea. At right are pain locations in cases of congestive dysmenorrhea.

before menstruation. Spasmodic dysmenorrhea generally disappears during the mid-twenties. Congestive pain may continue until menopause and may get worse with each successive pregnancy.

Asked how one distinguishes between the two types of pain, Dalton replies: "The vital question is, 'How do you know if your period is coming?' If the sufferer looks vague . . . or wonders why such a stupid question is being asked, she obviously does not get the warning symptoms diagnostic of congestive dysmenorrhea."[20]

Fifteen years ago, when my gynecologist suggested I try aspirin to relieve severe menstrual cramps, I thought she was being patronizing. I explained that I had already tried Darvon and codeine and *they* hadn't worked, so what could I expect from plain aspirin? . . . She insisted, I capitulated, and much to my surprise it was effective.

In 1972, a story appeared in the *New York Times*,[21] reporting the results of a Mayo Clinic study of painkillers. Darvon, said the article, is the painkiller most often prescribed in the United States. While it is designed to relieve pain, the Mayo study found that Darvon is only slightly more effective than a sugar pill! Aspirin, the report continued, was found to be more effective in relieving pain than codeine, phenacetin, or acetaminophen. These drugs were, however, more effective than Darvon, Zactane, or Sparine, the last three being only a little more effective than the placebo. The doctors who had conducted this investigation also pointed out that aspirin is much cheaper and has fewer side effects.

The women who answered the menstrual questionnaire gave the following list of proven remedies for menstrual pain:

Marijuana, sex, yoga, having a nice friend put his warm hands on my ovaries, peppermint tea (it works!), raspberry tea, a stiff drink, curling up with a heating pad, bone meal tablets, Alka Seltzer, Premarin, aspirin, a good shot of gin, seeing my lover smile. . . . The only medication I ever found that was effective was taken off the market. . . . The name of the medication was Edrisal.

A number of women have reported excellent results with Edrisal and so I called the FDA to ask why it was removed from sale. I was told that Edrisal contained amphetamine, aspirin, and phenacetin. All drugs that combine amphetamines and other agents were taken off the market in an attempt to control the prescription of amphetamines, which had gotten out of hand. A physician can, of course, write a prescription for the same amount of amphetamine and phenacetin that was contained in Edrisal as long as the prescriptions are filled separately.

In cases where menstrual pain persists despite the use of any of the treatments mentioned above, hormone treatment may be in order. In Dalton's view, spasmodic dysmenorrhea results from a hormone imbalance where there is too much progesterone in relation to estrogen. In cases like this, additional estrogen may relieve the cramps. Oral contraceptives are commonly prescribed under these conditions.

Congestive dysmenorrhea, again according to Dalton, results from too much estrogen in relation to progesterone. In these cases the birth control pill may make the pain *worse*. She recommends treatment with progesterone for all premenstrual symptoms, including congestive dysmenorrhea (see page 73).

A birth control pill prescribed to alleviate menstrual pain is no different from one prescribed for contraceptive purposes—the side effects are the same. You have to decide if it is worth it, knowing the risks involved.

Bleeding Abnormalities

Under normal conditions, variations in bleeding pattern are common. With so much variability, how can one decide when a bleeding irregularity is normal and when it demands medical treatment? The normal range of flow is from three to seven days. You might, therefore, think that an eight-day flow is a symptom of a problem which must be treated. If your physician did a blood test and found anemia resulting from the extra loss of blood, you would naturally receive treatment; but if you were not found to be anemic, you might be advised not to worry and to live with an eight-day period.

To some extent, then, the decision on treatment for a bleeding abnormality (a statistical abnormality) depends upon your physician's evaluation of the seriousness of the problem balanced against the expense of diagnosis and treatment. In many cases, bleeding abnormalities are treated *only* when they present a threat to health or when they are symptomatic of a more serious health problem.

The medical terms for various bleeding irregularities may refer to the suspected origin of the problem. *Metrorrhagia*, for example, is bleeding which falls outside the normal time of cycle (such as staining a week after the last flow has ended), when systemic malfunction is the suspected cause. *Menorrhagia* is uterine bleeding, resulting from systemic malfunction, which occurs at the anticipated time but lasts longer than seven days. The very same symptoms are called *dysfunctional uterine bleeding* when hormone disruption is the suspected cause.

Many women who use IUD's suffer from menorrhagia. Unless blood loss reaches hemorrhagic proportions and/or leads to anemia, it is generally considered a normal reaction to the presence of an IUD. For some women, however, the heavy flow is so annoying that they decide to change their method of contraception—whether or not the symptom is considered normal. One of the respondents to the menstrual survey reported that after IUD insertion her flow became very heavy but 250 mg. of Vitamin C every day brought the flow back to normal.

CAUSES

Menorrhagia and metrorrhagia can result from malnutrition, chronic iron deficiency, diseases of the blood, heart disease, growths in the reproductive organs, or IUD's. They may also be side effects of treatment for unrelated illnesses. Reproductive problems which lead to both menorrhagia and metrorrhagia are cervical polyps, pelvic inflammatory disease (P.I.D.), fibroid tumors, endometriosis or cancers of the uterus (cervix or endometrium). Although bleeding irregularities may be a symptom of cancer, they are usually traced to one of the other sources.

Cervical polyps are small benign growths of the cervix. In more than half the cases where women are found to have such polyps, bleeding is noticed after intercourse or douching. Minor surgery is all that is needed to remove the polyp and end the bleeding irregularity.

Almost 20 percent of all cases of irregular bleeding in women under forty are caused by pelvic inflammatory disease (P.I.D.). P.I.D. occurs when an infection started in the vagina or uterus travels into the Fallopian tubes and abdominal cavity. It can be extremely painful and, if left untreated for a long time, extremely dangerous. P.I.D. can result from complications following pregnancy, abortion, or miscarriage, or from inadequately sterilized instruments put into the uterus. It can also result from untreated or insufficiently treated venereal disease. Whatever its origin, P.I.D. is usually treated with antibiotics. Because the Fallopian tubes do not have an abundance of blood vessels, antibiotics (which travel through the bloodstream) take a long time to affect P.I.D. once the infection reaches the tubes.

Fibroid tumors are benign growths found within the body of the uterus. While it is estimated that one in every five women has fibroids, most of us are not aware of their presence. When they remain fairly small and do not cause bleeding they are likely to remain undetected. Since there is no evidence that fibroids become cancerous, their undetected presence is no reason for worry.

Estrogen is not believed to be a cause of fibroid development, but once the tumor exists, it does stimulate its growth. During menopause, when estrogen decreases, fibroid tumors often shrink. Naturally, if estrogen therapy is begun the tumors may enlarge.

Fibroids can cause uterine bleeding. If the bleeding is not profuse, a woman may find it acceptable. Even if it doesn't bother her, however, it is wise to correct the condition because uterine bleeding may also be a symptom of uterine cancer. (Fibroid-caused bleeding, especially in a postmenopausal woman, will be a confounding symptom for a physician who is watching for the possible presence of a cancer.)

In general, the physician will recommend dilation and curettage for a woman who has bleeding from fibroids. D & C's usually are done under general anesthesia and often require at least an overnight stay in a hospital. (This of course means that they cost a good deal of money and contribute to the high premiums paid out in health insurance.) The D & C procedure includes dilating the cervix, inserting a curette, and scraping the endometrial lining. (Bits of cervical tissue are also taken.) The extracted tissue is studied and if cancer is found, a hysterectomy will be scheduled at once. More often than not cancer is not the cause of the bleeding, although fibroids certainly may be detected.*

Hysterectomy should *never* be performed without prior diagnostic curettage. A gynecologist may recommend the operation as treatment for fibroids, but hysterectomy is major surgery—a great strain to the body. (It is also very expensive.) Furthermore, fibroids often shrink after menopause, and in many cases a premenopausal woman's condition should simply be watched. Fibroids are a common enough reason for hysterectomy, but the operation is too often performed without sufficient reason. By all means get a second opinion before agreeing to surgery for fibroids and be sure that the rationale for such an opera-

---

* Endometrial aspiration is an alternative to D & C which is now available in some communities; it is cheaper, safer, and requires no hospital stay, since it is performed in the doctor's office under local anesthesia. This method is an adaptation of the suction-curettage procedure used in abortion. According to Dr. Edward Stim, a New York gynecologist, the technique is successful in 90% of cases where diagnostic examination of the endometrium is required.

tion makes sense to *you*. The presence of fibroids in themselves does not indicate the need for a hysterectomy unless they are very, very large or are causing severe bleeding.

Uterine bleeding may also be a symptom of *cervical cancer*.* If cervical cancer is detected in its early stages, the recovery rate is high. The common means of diagnosis of cancer of the cervix is the Pap test, which should be routinely performed. The Pap test should be given once a year, and after one's thirties, twice a year. It is painless and inexpensive. (In some communities, Pap smears may even be available without cost.)

Cancer of the endometrium is rare in young women and peaks in frequency in the menopausal age range. Bleeding at irregular intervals may be the only symptom of this disease, but remember that this type of bleeding is usually caused by something far less serious. D & C or endometrial aspiration will be used to diagnose the source of bleeding, and hysterectomy will be recommended at once if cancer is detected. Either of these diagnostic procedures may also be therapeutic. Even if the source of the bleeding is never found, the bleeding usually clears up after the procedure.

Under normal conditions endometrial tissue only grows within the uterus. Sometimes, however, this tissue grows in other areas, causing *endometriosis*. The tissue behaves in the same way as the lining of the uterus; it builds up under the stimulation of estrogen, and bleeding takes place as estrogen is withdrawn. Endometrial tissue can grow on the ovaries, intestines, or abdominal cavity. Pain or irregular bleeding often accompanies the condition, which is frequently brought under control by hormone treatment.

Many cases of irregular menstrual flow are diagnosed as dysfunctional uterine bleeding.

> The premise that all abnormal uterine bleeding from the uterus in the absence of pregnancy, neoplasm, and inflammation is dysfunctional categorizes it but does not clarify its etiology. The subsequent deduction that it is, rather loosely, of endocrine origin . . . fails to decipher its origin. Nor does the use of such a "pedantic, pseudo-erudite expression" as dysfunctional uterine bleeding make us less ignorant of its cause-and-effect relationships. The immediate cause of dysfunctional uterine bleeding must remain a mystery as long as we are uncertain of the precise mechanism of the normal uterine bleeding—menstruation.[22]

---

* The incidence of cervical cancer parallels that of cancer of the penis. This has led doctors to believe that cancer of the cervix is sexually transmitted.

This kind of irregular bleeding is most common during the years when the hormone system is switching from one mode to another—the years after menarche and just before menopause. When it appears in young women, hormone therapy is often started without prior surgical diagnosis. In older women, hormone treatment is rarely started before a diagnostic curettage has been performed. As already mentioned, in 40 percent of the cases such curettage successfully stops the bleeding problem and no further medical attention is needed.

The normal range for onset of menstruation is from nine to seventeen years. If a young woman reaches eighteen and still has not begun menstruation, she is said to have *primary amenorrhea*. (A young woman may feel abnormal if she hasn't begun menstruating by the time she's sixteen, but as far as diagnosis is concerned she's still normal, and there's no need to pursue the matter medically.)

For this eighteen-year-old, however, a complete medical examination is in order. Almost half of the women with primary amenorrhea are found to have some genetic abnormality or a form of hermaphroditism. While these are rare conditions, the sooner they are detected, the sooner treatment can begin.

The fact that a critical weight and body composition must be reached before menstrual cycles begin means that for some young women primary amenorrhea may be the result of overly rigorous dieting. There is also a critical weight at the other extreme of the scale at which menstrual flow will be prevented. The degree of obesity that delays menarche is far greater than the degree of leanness that blocks the menstrual cycle.

Once menstruation has begun, the disappearance of cycles at any point between menarche and menopause (except of course during pregnancy) is called *secondary amenorrhea*. Among the many possible causes of secondary amenorrhea are disorders of nervous system functions, malfunctions of the pituitary or thyroid glands, disorders of the ovaries, psychological disturbance (as seen, for example, in cases of false pregnancy), and the use of oral contraceptive pills.

Dr. Rose Frisch has demonstrated that after menarche, a weight loss of 10 to 15 percent below the critical weight for maintaining cycles (an average of 121 pounds) can cause the loss of menstruation. This may explain why women who have gone overboard on crash diets, or those who have lost a lot of weight (and more particularly fat) on vegetarian, macrobiotic, or fruitarian diets, also lose the menstrual cycle. These diets may not in themselves be dangerous to health, but they may cause irregularity and then the complete suppression of ovulation and menstruation. If weight hovers around the point where menstruation stops, some cycles will be suppressed and others not. Again this is not in itself dangerous but may present problems if conception occurs. Children born to macrobiotic mothers tend to have a low birth weight; it has been demonstrated that underweight newborns have more health problems than those who are of average weight or above.*

We don't yet know enough about the long-term course of menstrual suppression as a result of lack of weight. It may be that long-term suppression leads to an inability to regain the menstrual cycle and fertility, even when body composition changes.

Any woman who has recently lost weight or has begun a new pattern of eating which has resulted in a loss of fat and has lost menstruation would easily be able to find out if menstrual suppression is caused by diet. Simply by eating more, and more high-caloric foods, the weight and fat would be regained and menstrual cycles would return. If diet is not the cause, the cycles will remain suppressed and medical attention is in order.

Cryptomenorrhea is a rare condition which only superficially resembles primary amenorrhea. Because of a blockage in the vagina or uterus, the young woman doesn't know she is menstruating. Menstruation occurs but the blood cannot escape. Minor surgery removes the block and flow appears.

Vicarious menstruation is an exceedingly rare condition in which cyclic bleeding occurs from a non-uterine source. Blood may come from the nose, eyes, or gastrointestinal tract. Mucous membrane is very responsive to estrogen, a fact we observe under more normal conditions when we experience nasal congestion or swelling before menstruation.

New Wives' Tales

For most of my life I have felt that there was something suspect about people who pay too much attention to exercise and eating

---

* This fact supports Dr. Frisch's hypothesis that critical weight is an adaptive mechanism. If the mother has an insufficient number of stored calories, her baby will be underweight. By cutting off fertility at a critical weight, fewer underweight babies are born.

habits.* My attitude has begun to change, however, and maybe this is my response to a change in attitude occurring in many people. Men and women are jogging up and down roads and around reservoirs; health food stores have sprung up in shopping malls and small towns. Women are discovering that eating well and exercising vigorously have positive effects on the experience of menstruation and menopause. I'm sure it is no coincidence that the women I know who have recently become menopausal have both exercised regularly and had few if any menopausal symptoms. I have noticed that when I ride my bike regularly and rely on it for transportation, I have almost no symptoms associated with menstruation.

Adelle Davis recommends that women with premenstrual distress take calcium every day, starting ten days to a week before they expect flow. (Calcium should be taken in conjunction with magnesium and Vitamin D.) Calcium, she tells us, is nature's tranquilizer, and the tension, irritability, and depression associated with menstruation and menopause may come from insufficient amounts of calcium. Many women have found this regimen effective. One of the respondents to the menstrual questionnaire wrote:

I start getting bitchy and snapping at my roommate about a week before my period. The first time that happens I start taking about 1½ grams of calcium lactate a day, which restores my disposition, and also helps prevent cramps. When I start bleeding, I raise the dose to 3 g per day. (K.K.)

Another woman reported the benefits of exercise and good eating habits:

When I began menstruating I also began formal dance training. As long as I kept in training I had no "physical distress." About five years ago I changed my profession. Now I'm no longer maintaining muscle tone as I did. I am suffering cramps. . . . I have noticed if I indulge my craving to stuff with food, my cramps are more severe. If I stay somewhat empty my cramps are mild—more nonexistent. (R.R.)

---

* A recent critical commentary to a pamphlet called *The Miracle of Living Foods* (Solana Health Center, Atlanta, Texas) provides this stunning guidance: "It is especially noteworthy that women who do not befoul their bodies with poison habits and dead food DO NOT MENSTRUATE! Hygienists have pointed this out for nearly a hundred years! Menstruation is symptomatic of inherent body pathology." In two sentences these people provide us with a complete misunderstanding of the relationship between diet and menstruation while at the same time reinforcing the worst prejudices of the menstrual taboo.

Some women even sent in diagrams to show the postures they find useful. One woman wrote about a problem of pain after intercourse which occurred during the premenstrual week:

Over a period of about a year I had very intense pains just after inter- course that would last 5 to 10 minutes. It seemed to happen usually during the week just before my period. I went to several doctors and they suggested: 1) it was gas; 2)I needed a psychiatrist. It was finally solved—the fourth doctor found the source of the problem. [The uterus had shifted position.]

Postures that may reduce menstrual pain. It has been suggested that posture d (on following page), when assumed shortly before intercourse, success- fully prevents postcoital pain

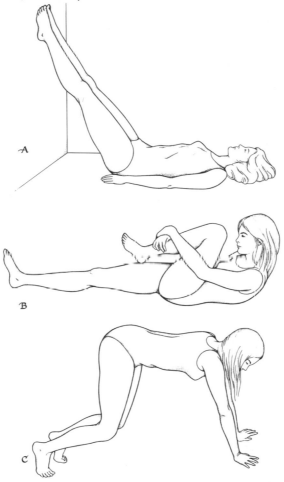

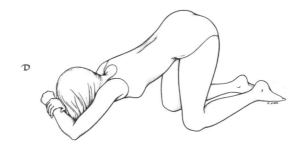

The solution was extremely simple. Kneel for five minutes before intercourse the week before my period. This completely solved the problem. [See illustration above.]

I mention it . . . because I had to undergo such humiliation and pain before a doctor happened to examine me while my uterus was flopped. There may be a lot of women with this kind of problem whose doctors recommend psychiatric help! (S.A.)

There is no doubt but that much more research into the causes and cures of menstrual and menopausal distress must be done. And there is no question that the lessening of the taboo surrounding these cycles of women's life will make our experience different and better. However, we don't have to suffer passively through menstruation and menopause. We can work for a change in research priorities and social attitudes, take good care of our bodies, and take advantage of those benefits which are already available—whether medical or not.

4

Taboo

The menstrual taboo is universal. "The notion that women's sexual processes are impure is worldwide and persistent," says Hays in *The Dangerous Sex*.[1] Menstrual blood is considered a volatile fluid capable of wide-ranging destruction; Pliny defines it as "a fatal poison, corrupting and decomposing urine, depriving seeds of their fecundity, destroying insects, blasting garden flowers and grasses, causing fruits to fall from branches, dulling razors. . . ."[2]

And the powers of menstrual blood are not confined to the world of the garden. "If the menstrual discharge," Pliny continues, "coincides with an eclipse of the moon or sun, the evils resulting from it are irremediable; and no less so when it happens while the moon is in conjunction with the sun; congress with a woman at such a period being noxious and attended with fatal effects to man."[3] Nor are its capabilities divorced from the woman who discharges this fluid once each month. According to Hays:

> The dangers of contact and contagion are so great that women are nearly always secluded or forced to reside apart during their monthly periods. Special huts are built for them by the Bakairi of Brazil, the Shuswap of British Columbia, the Guari of northern India, the Veddas of Ceylon and the Algonquin of the North American forest. From this it can be seen that the custom covers the globe.[4]

In cultures where a menstruating woman is not physically isolated, the taboo may take other forms, ensuring that she will do no harm. Frazer in *The Golden Bough* says:

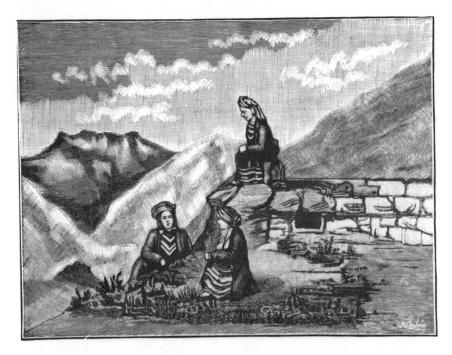

A menstrual hut in the Caucasus Mountains

A Native American menstrual hut

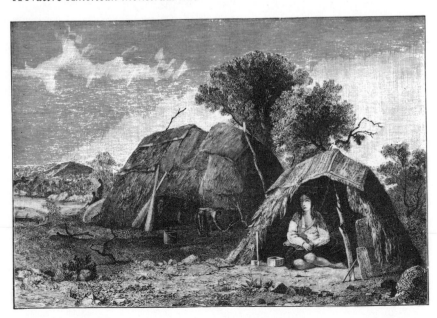

In Uganda, pots which a woman touches while the impurity of menstruation is upon her have to be destroyed; spears and shields defiled by her touch are, however, merely purified.

Among the Bribri Indians of Costa Rica the only plates she may use for her food are banana leaves, which when she has done with them, she throws away in some sequestered spot; for were a cow to find them, and eat them, it would waste away. And she drinks out of a special vessel for the same reason: if any one drank out of the same cup after her, he would surely die.[5]

Even this is not enough. Rules are made to purify the environment in cases where it is defiled:

. . . a sort of fumigating takes place. Siberian Samoyed women step over fires of burning reindeer skin.

Among the Dogan of East Africa the menstrual taboo is so strong that a woman in this condition brings misfortune to everything she touches. Not only is she segregated in an isolated hut and provided with special eating utensils, but if she is seen passing through the village a general purification must take place.[6]

In some cases punishment rather than purification becomes the focus for communities that wish to be protected from menstruating women. Among the ancient Persians (and in some outlying areas in contemporary communities), it was believed that menstruation lasts for four days. During this time women were kept apart in isolated huts and, in more recent times, in special rooms within the household. At the end of four days a woman who still menstruated was given one hundred lashes and sent back into seclusion for five more nights. At the end of this time if she continued to menstruate, she was given four hundred lashes because she was "possessed" by an evil spirit. Only then would purification measures begin. There have been societies which inflicted much more severe penalties, as Crawfurd points out: "Among the Australian blacks, the boys are taught from early childhood that if they set eyes on menstruous blood their hair will turn gray and their vigor abate prematurely. . . . The woman is forbidden under pain of death to touch anything that the men use or to walk on the paths they frequent."[7] And Novak adds: "The Illinois Indians punished with death any of their squaws who failed to give notice that they were affected by the periodic discharge."[8]

Not surprisingly, traditions evolved which enabled women who were not put into isolation to give fair warning that menstruation was in progress. Crawfurd goes on: "Among the people of the lower Congo . . . if a woman in this condition was to pass near some men who are likely to give her the equivalents of 'Good morning' or 'Good evening,' she will deliberately put her pipe in her mouth as a sign that she cannot answer because she is unclean."[9] Novak describes how, in Angola, "the women are obliged to wear a bandage about the head during the period of menstruation."[10]

In at least one culture, the powers of a menstruating woman were so virulent that they were believed to endure beyond her lifetime:

> In India the belief is widespread that a woman who dies during the prescribed period of her uncleanliness later lives as a ghost. . . . The Churel (ghost) is particularly harmful to its own family, but also to others. It appears in various forms. Usually it assumes the form of a beautiful young woman and leads men astray at night, especially those who are good looking. She takes them out of their realm into her own and keeps them there till they have lost their manly beauty. Then she sends them back into the world as gray-haired old men who find all their friends long dead.[11]

Blood and the Supernatural

In every case this taboo represents the fear and the supposition that menstrual blood contains supernatural powers. As Frazer describes it:

> The divine person who epitomizes the corporate life of his groups is a source of danger as well as of blessing: he must not only be guarded he must be guarded against. His sacred organism, so delicate that a touch may disorder it, is also, as it were, electrically charged with a magic or spiritual force which may discharge itself with fatal effect on whatever comes in contact with it. Hence the disastrous effect supposed to attend a breach of taboo; the offender has thrust his hand into a divine fire which shrivels and consumes him on the spot. . . .
>
> To seclude these persons from the rest of the world so that the dreaded spiritual danger shall neither reach them, nor spread from them, is the object of the taboos which they have to observe. These taboos act, so to say, as electrical insulators to preserve the spiritual force with which these persons are charged from suffering or inflicting harm by contact with the outer world.[12]

The taboo of menstruation does not preclude positive associations to this blood. Some reports of the beneficial effects of menstrual blood concern its properties as a medication. But one immediately suspects that this is another association of menstruation with disease, as in Pliny's claim that menstrual flow caused dogs to become rabid and cures the rabid dog's victim. Crawfurd reports that Ictidas, the physician, suggested that victims of quartan fever engage in sexual intercourse with a menstruating woman as a cure—although what effect this therapeutic measure had on the woman is left unsaid. In all events, the cases in which menstrual blood is used for good purpose are relatively few.

Generally, the object of a taboo may be a source of good or evil, but in the case of menstrual blood the ascriptions are almost universally evil. Another aspect is the belief that by secluding the person, he or she (as well as everyone else in the community) will be protected from the "divine" powers. Here again, however, the menstrual taboo is a most particular case of taboo: "Menstruating women are not a danger to themselves or to other women. . . . By far the dominant belief appears to be that menstruating women are dangerous to men."[13] The taboo is formulated to ward off such powers.

One might think that these beliefs and practices are the province of primitive peoples whose superstitions and conceptions of magic are quite literally more primitive and insubstantial than our own. One would be wrong.

The folk traditions of Western culture provide us with the beginnings of insight into contemporary belief:

> Gypsies believe that the witches have their sabbath on a Friday night on "Moon Mountain." They renew their pact with the devil once every seven years on such a mountain. During these seven years, Gypsy women collect their menstrual blood and, during the pact, they give all this blood to the devil to drink.
>
> It is believed that rocks seen on mountain tops, which turn red if water pours over them, are rocks where the devil spilled blood as he drank.[14]

One might also think that with the development of religions with which we are more comfortable, such beliefs would stop. Again, this is an incorrect assumption. In the traditions of those religions which replaced magical cults, the evaluation of menstruating woman remains identical with earlier versions:

> If in this state she will pollute mere man, still more will she pollute a sacred man. A menstruating Jewish woman was formerly forbidden to shake hands with a Rabbi, and women at these times were excluded from the Jewish synagogues and from the communion table of the early Christian Church.[15]

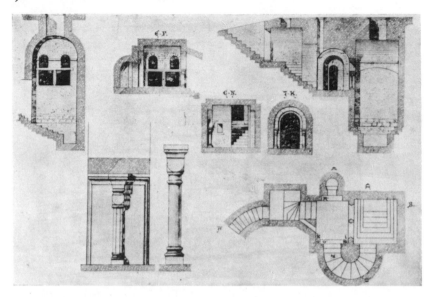

*Building plans for baths in which Jewish women of Worms and Rheims
performed ritual cleansing after each period of menstrual flow*

At the beginning of the twentieth century, Greek Orthodox
women were prohibited from taking communion when they were
menstruating. At a recent meeting of Native Americans, a medicine
man instructed any menstruating members of the audience to leave
the room before he began his prayers because the prayers would lose
all effectiveness in their presence.*

The ethical and moral beliefs on which contemporary religions are
based trace the evil of woman to menstruation and suggest that from
her evil all evil flows:

> The menstruous woman is possessed by an evil spirit; the spirit resides
> in her blood, and by the medium of her menstrual blood may exert its
> influence, for good or harm, or her environment. The evil spirit may
> affect its entry into the woman in the form of a bird, or a lizard or a
> serpent; hence the folk association of these animals with menstruation.
> It was the serpent that marred primordial bliss of Eden.[16]

The most damning euphemism attached to menstruation reflects
the belief that the monthly flow of blood is the curse God laid upon
woman for her sin in Eden. This is not an example of the misconcep-

---

* Contemporary religious practices are discussed in chapter 5 as they relate
to sexual activity, and in chapter 8 as they relate to woman's conception
of herself.

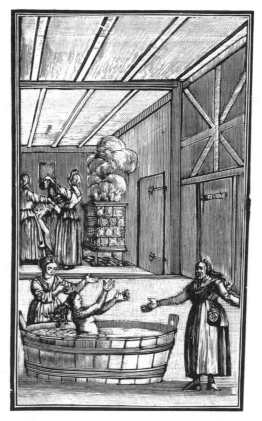

Tub bathing as a means of ritual purification among the Jewish women of Fürth

tions of the ancient past, but continues to carry the weight of belief, as Archie Bunker in *All in the Family* makes sure we understand:*

> *Archie*: Read your Bible. Read about Adam and Eve. . . . Going against direct orders, she makes poor Adam take a bite out of that apple. So God got sore and told them to get their clothes on and get outta there. So, it was Eve's fault God cursed women with this trouble. That's why they call it, what do you call it, the curse.[17]

In our culture, we do not consciously label menstruation evil, nor do we believe our taboo practices are based on this belief. For example, few who refrain from intercourse during menstruation think of this as protection against contamination by an evil spirit. Instead it is

---

* Copyright © 1973 by Tandem Productions, Inc. From the television show *All in the Family*, written by Michael Ross and Bernie West. In response to this statement another character used the word "menstruation," which resulted in a flood of critical mail.

called religious belief, a matter of preference, or aesthetics. Members of many of the tribes whose practices have been described above don't consider themselves to be "practicing" the menstrual taboo any more than we believe we are. It is a matter-of-fact part of life, not subjected to self-conscious scrutiny, as much a part of our culture as it is of all the other cultures. As Freud says, speaking of the taboo of virginity, "Wherever primitive man institutes a taboo, there he fears a danger; and it cannot be disputed that the general principle underlying . . . these regulations and avoidances is a dread of woman. . . . There is nothing in all this which is not still alive in the heart of man today."[18]

Sophisticated, literate modern-day men have the same fears as their primitive brothers had. These are fears held by men and directed toward women. No one imagines that a more noble emotion motivates the taboo, nor does anyone imagine that the taboo gains its generative power from women.

Stevens points out that men would rather have their wives present than sequestered in a hut, that they would prefer women to do the cooking rather than be barred from touching men's utensils, that they would presumably prefer to have sex than be prohibited from intercourse during the time of flow. But men have not acted out of this preference—they have made the choice to keep women separated during the time of flow, indicating the magnitude of the fear and the dimensions of danger they embody. Those men who have freely chosen to give up companionship, sex, and domestic service clearly have not felt the danger a trivial aspect of femininity.

The menstrual taboo exists as a method of protecting men from a danger they are sure is real (the source of which is in women), and it is a means of keeping the fear of menstruating woman under control. As soon as women succeed in overthrowing the taboo, these fears will no longer be comfortably contained. What is now covert may well become overt as male anxieties come to the surface. Because the taboo was instituted by men and because menstruation is considered a force which will, in general, only be harmful to men, a good deal of what is uncovered about the origins of the taboo will concern the nature of the male of the species—or at least an aspect of his nature which has thus far been carefully hidden.

The incest taboo affects the sexes in approximately equal fashion, and the destruction of the incest taboo would affect the sexes equally; but the menstrual taboo is the result of the fears of one sex about the other. The advantages and disadvantages of the taboo will therefore be appraised quite differently depending on one's sex. For men, the taboo actually reinforces their fears and keeps them from examining them but, in the immediate present, acts to reduce their anxiety.

For a woman, the taboo acts as a constant confirmation of a negative self-image. It represents the source of the shame she feels about her body and her sexuality. The moment she refuses to abide by the rules of the taboo, she will no longer be defined by its laws.

Of course, it is extremely hard to abandon these cultural laws. The belief that menstruation is dirty or, at the very least, unaesthetic is so deeply embedded that the opposite assertion, that it is beautiful, seems ridiculous. But the courage to be ridiculous is what is needed. Courage can be gained by joining with other women and by taking a closer look at the origins of the taboo involved.

Origins of the Taboo

What *is* the source of man's fears?

Margaret Mead[19] believes that the menstrual taboo can be traced to primitive man's fear of blood. Crawfurd expresses it, "Blood is the life," the spirit resides in blood. In the words of Hays, "Blood in all of its manifestations is a source of mana." And Frazer points out that:

> Some Indian tribes of North America ". . . abstain in the strictest manner from eating the blood of any animal, as it contains the life and the spirit of the beast." . . . Jewish hunters poured out the blood of the game they had killed and covered it over with dust. They would not taste the blood, believing that the soul or life of the animal was in the blood, or actually was the blood. The same belief was held by the Romans, and is shared by the Arabs, by Chinese medical writers and by some of the . . . tribes of New Guinea.
>   It is a common rule that blood may not be shed on the ground. . . . The reluctance to spill royal blood seems to be only a particular case of a general unwillingness to shed blood or at least let it fall on the ground. . . . [If] the soul is in the blood . . . any ground on which it falls . . . easily becomes taboo. . . .[20]

The supposition that the menstrual taboo is merely a subcategory of the blood taboo does not seem plausible. If all blood is a source of mana, why is it that men *and only* men consider menstrual blood identical in spiritual substance with other blood? What makes women's attitude toward blood so very different? How did women come to make the distinction between "life blood" and menstrual discharge?

Eventually we learn the relationship between the seriousness of the injury and the amount of blood. Children first connect "bigness" with importance, as the phenomenon of choosing the nickel over the dime amply proves. After a long time, I eventually understood that a lot of blood didn't mean that I was in mortal danger.

Later, when I went to school, I learned about another "kind" of blood. The blood of biology lessons wasn't something I could smell, touch, or even see. It took years before I believed that this second kind of blood really existed, although I immediately acted as though I believed the lesson at its first presentation.

At menarche, I learned a third lesson about blood. Unlike the first lesson, menstrual blood wasn't the result of an injury, and, unlike the second, it didn't stay inside the body—it could be smelled, touched, and seen. I don't know how long it took me to accept *this* lesson, but eventually I did. With regularity, menstrual flow would start, last for a few days, and then end.

Primitive peoples are preliterate peoples—they are not psychologically less developed than those of us who read and write. They are not victims of arrested development who are incapable of learning about the existence of natural events with repeated exposure. A woman who menstruates is perfectly healthy, and the regular reappearance of menstruation should make this lesson quite clear. There is nothing abstract about this experience, nothing that requires formal education to understand. Every woman learns the lesson of menstrual blood quite early in life and so might every man. The "primitive horror" of blood does not explain why menstruation must be taboo.

Men apparently have been unable to learn that menstrual blood is a natural event. They too might have seen it, touched it, and smelled it. But by choosing to make menstruation taboo, the power of menstrual blood to elicit terror was naturally increased. Freud adds:

> Other considerations, however, warn us not to exaggerate the influence of a factor such as a horror of blood. After all, the latter does not suffice to suppress customs like the circumcision of boys and the still more cruel extirpation of the clitoris and labia minora in girls . . . nor to abolish the prevalence of other ceremonies at which blood is shed.[21]

The fear of blood is not a sufficient explanation for still another reason, because the taboo has persisted into the present day when the horror of blood is no longer as great. Attitudes and feelings have

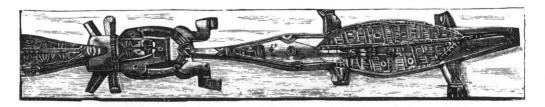

Wood carving from New Guinea depicting a woman whose head is held still by one crocodile while another crocodile extracts her menstrual flow

changed, yet each month when the blood flows from a woman's genitals the attitudes toward *it* remain unchanged.

The source of the taboo is powerful enough to override man's desire for a mate and a helper, and it is strong enough to override his capacity to learn by experience that the blood is a natural, normal occurrence. Again, the question must be posed: What is the source?

> The Negritos of the Malay Peninsula maintain there was once an ancestral creator, the monitor lizard. Since his contemporaries were all men, the lizard caught one of them, cut off his genitals and made him into a woman who became the lizard's wife and the ancestor of Negritos.
>
> . . . New Guinea carvings show images of women with a crocodile attacking the vulva, a hornbill plunging its beak into the organ or a penislike snake emerging from it.[22]

In cultures where the myths of creation center on a female figure as the creator, one doesn't expect to find the image of woman as a castrated man. However, where man or a male is named creator of the universe there must be some way of accounting for the anatomic "peculiarity" of the female. In many of these cultures, one might say the myths begin with the assumption that in the beginning was the penis.

When woman is mythically described as a castrated male, menstrual blood may be seen as the symbol of castration. The myths of male creation may reflect assumptions of a culture in which those who imagined creation already had power and projected it onto the mythic tale. As long as they retain this power, the myth remains alive. In this context, one wonders about the source of the menstrual taboo. After all, given that men already have power, the image of woman emerging by an act of castration might most naturally be the source of feelings of pity or superiority. Instead, the symbol of castration

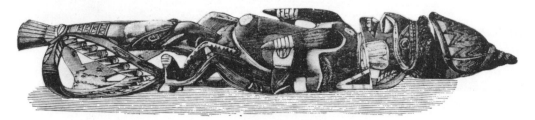

Wood carving from New Britain depicting a bird extracting menstrual blood from a woman's genitals

elicits dread. But woman is the castrated being, and what can harm man in that?

At this point, the search for the origins of taboo takes quite a turn. The myth that woman was created by the act of castrating a man, a thought not rationally explicable, is more plausibly explained as the result of man's projection of *his* fear of castration. The sight of blood coming from the female genitalia causes man anxiety because it forces to the surface his anxiety about male castration—the sign of which would be blood coming from *his* genitals. The creation myth of female birth through castration serves a dual purpose: It reasserts man's superiority (he still has his genitals intact), and it also calms his castration anxiety by making woman, not man, the victim.

The punishments meted out to men who break the rules attached to the menstrual taboo tend to support the idea that male castration anxiety plays a role in the genesis of the taboo. A common thread running through the taboos in many cultures is the belief that man will lose his potency if he comes in contact with menstruating woman. Reversing this logic, there is the belief that man will remain virile as long as he stays away from menstruating women.

If male fear of castration is the motive force behind the menstrual taboo, it must be demonstrated that this anxiety is as formidable today as it was thousands of years ago. At the simplest level, of course, the fact that male genitalia are external and exposed causes men to be vulnerable to injury and the possibility of castration. However, castration is an extremely rare occurrence, and one might wonder why anxiety about this unlikely event is and has been fierce enough to generate the menstrual taboo. Why didn't the fear of castration subside in the absence of reinforcement and the menstrual taboo created from it similarly disappear?

A look into contemporary mythology may supply at least a partial answer. Freud's mythic rendering of the creation of the psychic structure has colored our relationship to the world of the unknown. This has taken place in the absence of evidence that clearly confirms his hypotheses. Nonetheless, Freudian theory has permeated our culture and most of us are at least aware of the concept of castration anxiety which forms a part of it.

In the mythology developed by psychoanalysis, "the taboos represent an inculcated system of ego defense mechanisms."[23] The menstrual taboo, therefore, would represent the ego's defense from otherwise insupportable terror. What is the terror? If, as the male creation myths suggest, the source is fear of castration, then one must ask another question: Why is man in such a state of perpetual castration anxiety?

To find Freud's answer one must go to the analytic myth of the origins of civilization and psychic creation, since Freud believed that the fear of castration resulted from the actions which were responsible for the development of civilization. Elaborating on Darwin's theory that the earliest form of human social life was the horde, Freud postulated that precivilized men and women lived in small groups, called primal hordes, in which the dominant male controlled all the women and all the other men. The men who were not dominant, the sons of the leader of the horde, had sexual access to women *only* when the father chose to give permission. The sons reacted to this situation with rage and frustration which eventually reached proportions that could no longer be controlled. Freud next hypothesized that the sons developed a plan through which they could seize access to the women. If they acted collectively they could overpower the father, kill him, and take control of the women, and this they did.

However, in order to prevent a repetition of the tyranny of the primal fathers, the sons realized that they must make some rule to prohibit any one man from sexually possessing all women. The incest taboo was created, which limited the sexual relations between man and woman. The primal sons astutely perceived what Freud thousands of years later succinctly observed: "Sexual desires do not unite men, but divide them."[24]

"In the beginning," Freud quotes from Goethe, "was the deed."[25] The deed in his view was murder of the primal father. Although the sons gained sexual freedom through this deed, the analytic myth explores quite a different result as well: the sons experienced enormous guilt for their act of patricide.

An ancient Indian myth which seeks to explain the origins of menstruation provides an interesting illumination of Freud's point:

> A queen whose daughter was menstruating asked her husband, "Lord, tell me, you who know the nature of things, how women came to menstruate? How it happened in the old days that it still remains today?" The king answered her: "Once Indra killed the demi-god Visvarupa . . . with his powerful thunderbolt. He killed him in battle. He returned to his dwelling but reaped no fame. Instead, Brahmatya, the personification of the murder of Brahmins, came to the god with folded hands and full of humility. Indra was afraid of her, and having been seized with fear he felt no joy. The earth and all creatures called him a Brahmin murderer and Indra, tormented by Brahmatya, thought in his heart, 'What must I do to be free from the shame of this murder?' "

He first went to the Earth and persuaded the Earth to relieve him of part of his guilt. "He bowed before the Earth and gave part of his guilt. . . . The second part of this guilt, Indra gave to the streams." The third part the rocks and streams must share:

> "After he had thus given away three parts of his guilt, he spoke to the beautiful ones. His hands folded and full of humility, saying, 'Son, son (I am of you), take the fourth part of my guilt. You must not be negligent.'
>
> "When they all declared themselves agreeable, he spoke the following words to the long-eyed women bringing them the fourth part, 'Every month you admirable ones shall menstruate. For three days you shall not be touched. . . . Thereafter your life shall be completed.'
>
> "After the thousand-eyed one had bestowed this mercy upon them, he went forth to heaven. Freed from murder he now lived happily. From then on women have menstruated every month and, therefore, the woman is impure for three days in all her actions."[26]

This myth lends some support to Freud's elaboration of the primal crime. Freud, like the maker of the Indian myth, believed that insupportable guilt followed the act of murder. In the ancient Indian myth, the punitive force is represented by a female god and in the modern-day Freudian myth by the memory of the father's godlike power. In describing the way the murderer deals with his guilt, the ancient and modern myths sharply diverge. The ancient myth depicts a man who unburdens himself by placing a portion of his guilt on woman-the-mother. By projecting this guilt (in the form of the menstrual "impurity"), the male is liberated. In Freud's elaboration of the primal crime, however, projection doesn't exist.

In Freud's opinion the murderer remembers that while he lived, the primal father punished his sons by castrating them, killing them, and then eating them. After the primal crime the sons lived with the fear that they would be castrated in retaliation. In the beginning, Freud suggests, was the act of murder, the development of the incest taboo, and the fear of castration—the punishment which would fit the crime. Civilization developed from these foundations, and through racial memory we inherit the unconscious structures which perpetuate civilization and this basic fear.

The history of an individual recapitulates the history of the race. As Freud believed, the development of each boy recapitulates the beginnings of civilization. The Oedipus complex, which Freud believed universal, describes the boy's desire sexually to possess his mother, the wish to kill his father in order to remove the powerful obstacle to the mother, and the terror that he will be castrated for punishment of this *wish* as he would certainly be for the deed.

In the Freudian perspective, every man born since the dawn of civilization passes through the Oedipal stage of development and relives the depth of desire and hatred experienced by the sons of the primal horder. Every man, therefore, also has the anxiety that he will be castrated because his wishes make him deserving of castration.

In the Freudian myth of the primal horde, woman is a shadow. We know little about her nature. Presumably she had no vested interest in the rule of the primal father nor in the actions of the sons. In this myth, woman was a passive creature even *before* civilization began.

While woman remains a shadow, certain critical assumptions are made about her nature. In Freud's opinion, she too suffers from castration anxiety. In her case, however, this is not the result of guilt over the primal crime (in which presumably she had no role) but comes instead from her belief that originally she possessed a penis.* When woman realizes that she has been castrated, she becomes enraged. Eventually she comes to believe that by sexual union with

---

* Women in psychoanalytic treatment have contributed material that supports the concept of penis envy. One argues not with the "fact" of penis envy but with its interpretation. Freud accepted the idea that women believe they initially had a penis, lost it, and suffer as a result of this loss. (This suffering gives rise to the complex of penis envy.) Even if this were true, penis envy would only be the equivalent of womb or birth envy in men. (Freud ignored the latter; within his own framework he was lax.)

One might suspect that in cultures where the mother goddess reigned, women believed that in the beginning was the vagina/clitoris and that the first men grew penises—a biological development with some rather pleasurable implications for heterosexual enjoyment but hardly a monumental "advantage" to which envy is the "natural" response.

her father and by bearing the child that results she may gain a substitute for her lost penis.

After the primal crime, the incest taboo was developed by the sons. Woman was no longer permitted to have intercourse with her father, and the compensation for the missing penis was no longer available. Again, she experienced monumental rage, which diminished as she came to believe that the child of any other union could be her penis substitute.

Each girl child passes through a stage in which she realizes that she has been castrated and comes to desire her father and his child. She is forbidden to act this out, and her rage—first at being castrated, and then at being prohibited from having the best substitute for a penis— is repressed.

With respect to castration both male and female psychic developments bear upon the menstrual taboo. Freud believed along with Frazer that taboos are instituted as a result of ambivalence and that the object of taboo is also the object of strong desire. If it were not desirable by nature, there would be no need to make a law forbidding relations with it. It may be presumed that man initially found menstruating woman desirable but had reason to outlaw actions based upon this lust. Indeed, Freud quite clearly states his belief in the motives for the taboo on women: "The strange taboo of virginity— the fear of which among some primitive peoples induces the husband to avoid the performance of defloration—finds its full justification of this hostile turn of feeling."[27]

According to Freud, in her reproductive crises (menarche, menstruation, menopause, the termination of virginity, and childbirth), woman's fury about the loss of a penis and the impossibility of union with her father surfaces. And, he concluded, the taboo is wisely constructed to protect man from his lust for this "demonic creature" who will definitely vent her rage upon him.

Freud, then, believed that banishing a woman from sight, forbidding her to touch utensils shared with man, or prohibiting sexual relations between man and menstruating woman are rational actions that men must take to protect themselves. The menstrual taboo spares man from witnessing the rage of woman's castration anxiety, and from being reminded of his own castration anxiety, which would be elicited by the sight of genital bleeding.

In *Totem and Taboo*, Freud acknowledged that he had given only a rough sketch of the possible origins of civilization. However, those who have followed him have adhered to his theory and his opinion

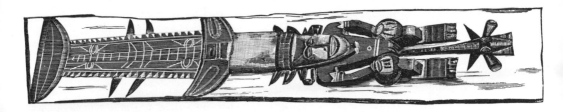

Wood carving from New Guinea in which a woman holds her thighs while a snakelike being emerges from her vagina

that menstruating woman is a demon and menstruation quite properly tabooed.

Another analyst who took this theoretical framework one step further is the British psychoanalyst C. D. Daly, a young contemporary of Freud's. While he accepted most of Freud's theoretical opinions, his self-analysis led him to reconsider the origins of the menstrual taboo. Agreeing with Freud's observations, Daly suggested that during menstruation woman feels exceptionally sexual.* He inferred that in the time of the primal horde, man found menstruation sexually exciting.

The incest taboo was initiated after the primal crime; if woman's sexuality was heightened during menstruation and the male's desire for her was also heightened, the emerging social order—the incest taboo—would be threatened:

> The sexual prerogatives of the primal males which had been normal to the horde phase passed away and the leaders of the tribes which replaced the hordes ruled with their powers considerably restricted. At the same time, in order to make the prohibition of incest effective, the young males . . . were threatened with castration. . . . Similarly, the females were isolated and starved and treated with endless cruelty. The prohibition of incest could hardly have been operative except by some such methods of collective cruelty.[28]

Daly's interpretation—that males were threatened with castration and, when menarche appeared, young girls subjected to cruel treatment to ensure the continuation of the incest taboo—presupposes the existence of active females who were able to exercise their desires and who consequently were banished in order to prevent them from so

---

* There is ample evidence to support Daly's contention that women do experience an increase in sexual desire at the time of menstruation—see chapter 5, p. 121.

doing. Although there is no reason to assume that Daly had knowledge of Amazonian mythology, the Tukano Indian legend of the Daughter of the Sun offers a perfect example of the point he made. According to the anthropologist Gerardo Reichel-Dolmatoff, the following ancient myth continues to play a role in present-day Tukano religious belief:

> The Daughter of the Sun had not yet reached puberty when her father made love to her. The Sun committed incest with her at Wainambí Rapids and her blood flowed forth; since then, women must lose blood every month in remembrance of the incest of the Sun and so that this great wickedness will not be forgotten. But his daughter liked it and so she lived with her father as if she were his wife. She thought about sex so much that she became thin and ugly and lifeless. . . . But when the Daughter of the Sun had her second menstruation, the sex act did harm to her and she did not want to eat any more. She lay down on a rock, dying; her imprint there can still be seen on a large boulder at Wainambí Rapids. When the Sun saw this, he decided to make *gamú bayári*, the invocation that is made when girls reach puberty. The Sun smoked tobacco and revived her. Thus, the Sun established customs and invocations that are still performed when young girls have their first menstruation.[29]

This legend might be used to corroborate Daly's contention that the taboo of menstruation developed from the need to curb incestuous desires. It further supports Daly's thesis that the female becomes the source of blame while the fears, pleasures, and culpability of males are ignored.

> For man, menstruous woman is taboo because this deeply unconscious id-attraction [to the menstruating woman] is associated with the unconscious ego's fear of being eaten and castrated, fear through which his incestuous desires were frustrated. Moreover, the previous hatred and fear of the father have been displaced onto woman, thus increasing her black magic. The terribly beautiful and loathsomely ugly aspects of the aggressive goddesses and witches have their genesis here.[30]

In his analysis of the origins of the menstrual taboo, Daly contributes two important elements overlooked or ignored by Freud: Woman feels intensely sexual during menstruation; and man, originally attracted to menstruating woman, projected his feelings toward the primal father onto her. Within the framework created by Freud, the father of psychoanalysis is shown to have had a critical blind spot—he had great difficulty in considering woman a person of substance.

In recent years many women have objected to Freud's mythology, claiming that he was bound by the repressive Victorian culture in which he lived. They contend that Freud did not describe the female psyche but instead presented a detailed description of the social position in which women lived. (Penis envy, according to these critics, represents woman's envy of male power and not, as Freud suggested, the aftermath of her supposed castration.)

When Freud suggests that a woman is in a state of rage during menstruation, he might simply be creating an elaborate psychic explanation for the rather straightforward repression of sexuality in the nineteenth century. To the extent that we subscribe to his mythology and to the premise which is its basis (that there is a definable psychic substratum which shapes all human experience), the meaning of the menstrual taboo is of considerably more than academic interest. If, for example, Freud is correct in his interpretation of the taboo, women have the responsibility for understanding and transcending an extreme emotional state (castration rage) if the taboo is to disappear. If the critics are correct, the taboo merely reflects the cultural downgrading of women. However, if Daly's suggestion is correct, or at least closer to the truth, men will confront serious emotional difficulty when women refuse to honor the taboo.

In her book *Psychoanalysis and Feminism*, an interpretation of analytic theories, Juliet Mitchell argued that the feminist criticism of Freud is unjust. Women may well resent the concept of penis envy, as we may well resent Freud's analysis of the menstrual taboo, but Freud brilliantly mapped the structure of the psyche which has existed in all patriarchal societies. We can hardly blame Freud, she explains, for the development of patriarchy; we may strenuously object to the role of women in patriarchal cultures, yet he was merely delineating it, not creating it.

> Men enter into the class-dominated structure of history while women (as women, whatever their actual work in production) remain defined by the kinship patterns of organization. In our society the kinship system is harnessed into the family—where a woman is formed in such a way that she will stay. Differences of class, historical epoch, specific social situation alter the expression of femininity; but in relation to the law of the father, women's position across the board is a comparable one. When critics condemn Freud for not taking account of social reality, their concept of that reality is too limited. The social reality that he is concerned with elucidating is the mental representation of the reality of society.[31]

Mitchell has successfully answered the critics of Freudian theory who have labeled him culture-bound. However, she has not successfully pinpointed Freud's blind spot. Freud himself was aware of the weakness in his mythology in dealing with the role of women. He spoke in *Totem and Taboo* of his failure to elaborate upon or analyze the role of the maternal deities, and as late as 1933, in the *New Introductory Lectures*, he admitted that woman remained a riddle to him, again calling attention to his lack of understanding.

To ignore Freud's weakness here is dangerous because the oversights and riddles in his theories are more than minor gaps in a brilliant analytic structure. If these gaps represent missing material of substance, as Daly's work amply indicates, then the puzzle put together by Freud must be drastically altered to make room for these "few outstanding bits." The pieces of the puzzle Freud uncovered will in many cases remain, but once the full dimension of female psychology is perceived, the configuration of the overall image will be completely different.

The concepts of penis envy and the child substitute, for example, contain large gaps, since the meaning of the mother goddesses has not yet been worked out. When this material is added to the psychoanalytic and anthropological reports of woman envy among males, the placement of penis envy and the child substitute in female psychology will be quite different.

The notion that the first woman was a castrated male and that quite "naturally" women themselves perceive their lack is substantiated by the creation myths in which a male god was the creator. This is the case where a lizard-god castrated a male to make his mate, a man-god took a rib from his human image to make woman, and a group of sons created civilization by an act of patricide.

If, however, a woman is the mythic creator of the world, there is no presumed initial lack of a generative or sexual organ. She gives birth to the world and to men and their mates. These myths do not lead to assumptions of penis envy with the child as compensation. As Frazer points out:

> . . . among the Khasis of Assam, the ancient system of mother-kin in matters of inheritance and religion is preserved to this day. For among these people the propitiation of deceased ancestors is deemed essential to the welfare of the community, and of all their ancestors they revere most the primaeval ancestress of the clan. Accordingly, in every sacrifice a priest must be assisted by a priestess; indeed, we are told that he merely acts as her deputy, and that she is without doubt a survival

of the time when, under the matriarchate, the priestess was the agent for the performance of all religious ceremonies.[32]

If civilization did not begin with patriarchy but rather with matriarchy, our psychic inheritance must include both the substance of feeling of matriarchal times and the acts by which matriarchy was overturned. We may at the very least suspect that in the beginning there was not penis envy but rather woman envy.

> There is a Persian myth of the creation of the world which precedes the biblical one. In that myth a woman creates the world, and she creates it by the act of natural creativity which is hers and which cannot be duplicated by men. She gives birth to a number of sons. The sons, greatly puzzled by this act which they cannot duplicate, become frightened. They think, "Who can tell us, that if she can *give* life, she cannot also *take life*." And so because of their fear of this mysterious ability of woman, and of its reversible possibility, they kill her.[33]

Here Frieda Fromm-Reichmann and her colleague Virginia Gunst consider the responses of men in this myth of woman creation; but surely the feeling of woman envy is part of the development of this emotion. She can do something which they cannot, and this alone is both insupportably blessed and terrifying.

The envy and fear of woman present in this early myth suggest a female psyche in which genital pride is far more real than genital envy—among women. It is not an isolated instance, as the noted psychologist Bettelheim shows:

> While men speak of the secret of women and mean their sex apparatus and functions, women do not make a similar association to the secrets of men. They may even scoff at the very idea of men's secrets. Berndt, in discussing the origin of the Australian Kunapipi [fertility] rites, refers to one of the myths that tells how originally, men "had nothing: no sacred objects, no sacred ceremonies, the women had everything." Or as one of Berndt's present-day informants told him: "But really we have been stealing what belongs to them, for it is mostly all woman's business; and since it concerns them it belongs to them. Men have nothing to do really, except copulate, it all belongs to the women . . . the baby, the blood, the yelling, the dancing, all that concerns the women; but every time we have to trick them."[34]

Bettelheim also discusses another tribe, the Changa, in which the males believe that menstrual blood has great power. The men are envious of this power and in an attempt to reduce their envy, they tried to gain equal power through a form of mimicry. They developed an initiation ceremony in which a plug is put into the anus. After initiation, they assert the existence of a unique male biological capacity—they no longer need to defecate. The men take care never to defecate where a woman might see them, so that no woman will ever learn that the "secret" power is a simple trick.

> The pretended stopping up of the anus has an additional meaning. It is not only connected with menstruation but also with pregnancy. Thus, the setting of the plug also imitates the stop in menstruating—that is the first indication of pregnancy. The Changa women, who are aware of what is going on, regard the men's behavior with amused tolerance. In their own initiation rites, the girls are told that the men defecate but keep it secret from the women, and they are admonished not to laugh. The women realize that actually the secret is theirs; they say that when a woman becomes pregnant her source of blood is stopped up and that this is the original plug.[35]

The Changa women, it would seem, were much closer to self-awareness than we are. While American women have been known to take secret pleasure in their "powers," this has been the meekest and least rewarding form of compensation for lack of self-esteem and power. Perhaps the sharpest definition of our diminished opinion of woman's worth is demonstrated by the feelings we harbor about menstruation and menopause. If these are indeed the true wonders, and men have wrested them from us, we have capitulated to men and come to accept the "natural" horror of menstruation and the downgrading of menopause.

In this connection, it is enlightening to examine the most direct example of woman envy and one which is most startling because it runs counter to every assumption about the negative meaning of menstruation.

Sub-incision rituals have been documented as a part of the ceremonial life of some tribes in New Guinea, Australia, the Philippines, and Africa. During these rites, says Bettelheim, surgery is performed on the penis:

> The operation consists essentially in slitting open the whole or part of the penile urethra along the ventral or under surface of the penis. The initial cut is generally about an inch long, but this may subsequently be enlarged so that the incision extends from the glans to the root of the scrotum; in this way the whole of the under part of the penile urethra is laid open. The latter form of the operation is universal among the Central tribes [of Australia]. As one proceeds outwards, the intensity of the operation becomes reduced, until we meet with forms

in which a small slit is made in the urethra towards either the glans or the scrotum, or both.[36]

Bettelheim goes on to make the point that the men perform sub-incision rituals in order to make the penis the equivalent of the female genitals. He cites the work of anthropologists who stated that in certain tribes of New Guinea the word for the introcised penis is the same as the word meaning "the one with a vulva." Anthropologists have also reported that among the Wogeo of New Guinea, men believe that menstruation is a cleansing process, and, wishing themselves to be clean, they "periodically incise the penis and allow some blood to flow; an operation which is often called 'man's menstruation.'"

> The Murgin say: "The blood that runs from an incision and with which the dancers paint themselves and their emblems is something more than a man's blood—it is the menses of the old Wawilak women. . . . 'That blood we put all over those men is all the same as the blood that came from the old woman's vagina. It isn't the blood of those men anymore because it has been sung over and made strong. . . .'"[37]

It is hard to imagine a more dramatic example of woman envy or of the principle of cultural relativity. Obviously menstruation is *not* universally believed to be a curse, although it may be that menstruation is universally envied. This, however, was lost to early psychoanalytic theorists.

Devereux has said that: "The menstruating woman as a witch is, in a sense, the central theme of the psychoanalytic approach to menstruation."[38] The analytic view, if not culturally bound, must be the result of an inability to see clearly. If man was not always the powerful figure he is in analytic mythology, and we have seen this demonstrated, then the nature of female psychology and most certainly of menstruation is not what the witch hunters found.

Mary Jane Sherfey, a psychoanalyst and author of *Nature and Evolution of Female Sexuality*, re-examined cultural history and postulated the existence of powerful women living before the time of the rise of patriarchy. While this idea might have given rise to theory which deviates from Freud's, Sherfey concludes that it merely substantiates his view that men were quite right to fear woman-power:

> There are many indications from the prehistory studies in the Near East that it took perhaps five thousand years or longer for the subjugation of women to take place. All relevant data from the 12,000 to 8,000 B.C. period indicate that precivilized women enjoyed full sexual freedom and were often totally incapable of controlling their sexual drives.

Therefore, I propose that one of the reasons for the long delay between the earliest development of agriculture (c. 12,000 B.C.) and the rise of urban life and the beginning of recorded knowledge (c. 8,000–5,000 B.C.) was the ungovernable cyclic sexual drive of women. Not until these drives were gradually brought under control by rigidly enforced social codes could family life become the stabilizing and creative crucible from which modern civilized man could emerge.[39]

Sherfey makes two assumptions in this statement which are questionable. First, by equating the era in which women were powerful with "precivilization," she is making an editorial judgment rather than stating a fact. Freud, after all, declared that civilization began with the primal murder in the days long, long before recorded history. The second assumption, that woman's sexuality was out of control, Sherfey herself modifies in a footnote: "However, I must make it clear that the biological data presented support only the thesis on the intense, insatiable eroticism in women."[40]

These women were not necessarily living before the dawn of civilization, nor were they necessarily an impediment to the development of civilization simply because they were intensely erotic—or even insatiable. It is by no means logically necessary to conclude that men *had* to subjugate women in order to get on with the business of building civilization. Given the same data, in fact, one could as easily postulate that man subjected woman to the oppression of the menstrual taboo because of moral lassitude. By "desexing" woman he would no longer have to deal with the profound confusions created in a world where everyone is sexual, and he would be spared the largest part of sexual competition with other men. The relationship between male sexual competition and menstruation is illuminated in the following myth of the Sinaugolo of New Guinea, quoted in Ploss and Bartles:

> In the old times the moon lived on earth as a young man of very tiny size and he was covered on his whole body with light colored hair. It was his habit to follow the women and girls to the garden.
> For a long time none of them paid any attention to him, until one day he began to scream, whereupon a married woman lifted him up and set him in her woven basket that hung on a limb. (According to another version, he himself climbed into a basket and from here he started to cry.) Then the woman told him to be quiet, she would fetch food for him and cook it.
> While she was digging out a yam root for this purpose, the little one slipped out of the basket and broke off a piece of sugar cane and

ate it. Thereupon he cohabited with the woman, with the result that she became pregnant.

Her husband accused her of adultery with the boy. Although she denied it, he was nevertheless suspicious and lay in wait for her. In a short time the pair came together, whereupon the youth climbed back into his basket which now hung in the garden-house, and here he again started to cry.

The woman said he should be quiet, she would give him to eat and then go back to the village. Her husband, however, lit a fire in front of the house and behind it so the boy was unable to escape and was killed.

His blood squirted up to heaven and here turned into the moon. The moon announced that in retribution all girls and young women shall bleed when he appears, but old women and pregnant ones are excepted, the latter since he was responsible for their condition.[41]

In this myth, the young man who becomes the moon does not respond to his murder by punishing the jealous husband who committed the crime. Instead, he punishes *all* women with the "curse." Menstruation, then, in terms of the myth of the Sinaugolo, is woman's punishment for a crime she did not commit, as was also the case in the ancient Indian myth cited earlier.

The sexually free woman, completely possessed neither by her husband nor her lover, becomes the alleged cause of a murder—the real cause of which was man's sexual jealousy. By penalizing *her*, one presumes, the equilibrium between men was restored, since both the boy-moon and the man-husband are satisfied that justice has been done once she is "cursed."

One might stretch the meaning of this myth and say that it proves that woman's insatiable sexuality needed forcible restraint. However, there is nothing that we have seen which logically compels us to make this assumption. The "curse" of menstruation is not the *inevitable* outgrowth of a need to curtail uncontrollable female sexual liberty. The taboo may well have resulted from man's decision to retain sexual freedom for himself, limit it in woman, and minimize sexual competition among men. This is a far less morally demanding choice for men since it requires no profound confrontation with the dilemma posed by passion. It is a choice that has crippled the freedom (sexual and otherwise) of half the members of our species.

In 1932 Mary Chadwick wrote a monograph on the psychology of menstruation. She explored the connection between sexual repression and the fear of menstruating woman. In her analysis of the taboo she found a link between the early religions that worshiped the mother goddess and the later corruptions of these religions found in witch cults. She speculates:

> Should we now examine carefully the history of witch-craft from the various sources of information that are available, we cannot help feeling that we find in them evidence enough to supply the theory that the witch-woman was to a great extent the menstruating woman.[42]

Her discussion of the motives which led to the persecution of witches can, by her own hypothesis, be extended to the motivations which result in the taboo of menstruation:

> The witch-cult is essentially a projection of repressed sexual wishes. . . . The fear and dread . . . of the witches was formerly caused, in all probability, by this same identification of the witch with the mother who might be dangerous and therefore must be killed by proxy. In this way the witch hunters of the middle ages would have the unconscious dynamic of mother hatred to add enthusiasm to their work, seeing in these women those who might even destroy them, if they didn't exterminate them first.[43]

Gregory Zilboorg is another critic who, in retracing the mythic steps leading to the origins of civilization, found the Freudian myth of creation lacking and its discussion of women androcentric. In his work, Zilboorg uses the writing of Lester Ward. Like Freud, Ward employed Darwinian theory to trace the emergence of human social life, but he came to a quite different interpretation of history:

> Primitive woman, though somewhat smaller, physically weaker, and esthetically plainer than man, still possessed the power of selection, and was mistress of the kinship group. Neither sex had any more idea of the connection between fertilization and reproduction than do animals, and therefore, the mother alone claimed and cared for the offspring, as is done throughout the animal kingdom below man. So long as this state of things endured the race remained in the stage . . . of female rule. That this was a very long stage is attested to by a great number of facts.[44]

Zilboorg and Ward point to a bitter irony contained in the pathways of human sexual selection: by exercising sexual choice, women gave birth to men who grew progressively larger and stronger; because of the far greater size and strength of men, the primal act became a reality. Zilboorg's view of the primal act was quite different from Freud's. In his opinion, the act was rape of the mother:

> The first cultural act and the first sexual act which led to the formation of a family were identical—the successful physical, narcissistic, sexual assault on woman. Perhaps it is here that one ought to look for the

sources of that controversy, cultural or sexual, which has been raging in and around psychoanalysis and confusing the real issues. The first economic and the first sexual self-assertion of the male were one and the same act; the family and the later cultural institutions were born from that explosive self-assertion. Man was unable to maintain the advantages he had momentarily gained through this act, unless and until he resolved his rivalry with the primordial mother by way of projecting onto her a good part of his own sadism as well and perhaps particularly by way of his identification with the mother.[45]

In Zilboorg's reconstruction of the creation myth, the subjugation of woman followed the primal crime. Only after the mother was raped and scorned did the male-dominated culture take shape. The control of sexual selection was taken from her, and in order to enforce man's newly won powers, he projected onto her the witchlike attributes we find in the menstrual taboo.

Zilboorg's mythology leads directly to quite different conclusions from Freud's. The racial inheritance of woman is rage resulting from the primal rape: it would not result in the major complex of penis envy but in rape anxiety. The threat of rape, deeply engrained in woman's psyche, would be one of the reinforcements of the menstrual taboos. Woman had best bend to man's projections and believe that menstruation is unclean and woman corrupt, because if she does not she will be brutalized. And unlike male castration anxiety, rape anxiety is all too often reinforced by the reality of the act of rape.

Psychologically and pragmatically the primal crime is re-created, and the results of it are seen in contemporary society—rape, denigration of women, and usurpation of woman's power. The psychological and practical implications of the primal crime of rape are further elaborated when we examine the economic results: "Women may be considered chronologically the first piece of property, in the true sense of the word, in that sense which Ward defined with unique simplicity and brilliance: Property is possession beyond one's immediate needs. It was possession beyond his immediate purely sexual needs that man established over woman."[46]

If the fear of rape is the unconscious horror which each girl child inherits, the birth into the station of property is the means by which the role of woman is solidified with finality. As long as woman is dependent upon man and as long as she fears the repetition of the primal rape as the punishment for her powers, she is likely to accept man's claim that her body is unclean.

Freud's mythology would have us believe that woman *is* unclean, that her rage over a lost penis has damned her, and that man must at all costs protect himself from this rage. Although one would not expect to find millions of women easily acknowledging Freud's hypothesis, it is almost impossible to meet *any* woman for whom his theory resonates with psychic truth.

Daly's hypothesis, because it is based on the idea that most women experience menstrually related sexual feelings quite naturally each month, has greater plausibility. Perhaps the need to suppress the sexuality of both sexes was a cornerstone for the building of civilization. This need, however, does not sufficiently explain the one-sided shape given to this repression. Perhaps, as Daly suggests, castration anxiety among men offers the missing motive. Menstruation must be taboo if man is to be saved the castration anxiety present in his psychic structure because he inherits the guilt of the primal murder. However, this does not substantially flesh out the shadow of woman. Man's castration anxiety, even when combined with the incest taboo, does not tell us why women have for so long accepted the definition incorporated in menstrual taboos.

Zilboorg's mythology, however, presents us with the first detailed reconstruction of a creation myth which meshes with the psyche of contemporary women. The rape of the primal mother and the devaluation of women that followed it are, for women, more plausible psychic maps than the murder of the primal father. Men, in the beginning, envied women and feared them. In the end, women fear men, but they do not envy them.

Woman's fear and dependency form the underpinnings of her current and historical role. The menstrual taboo which most plausibly arose from man's envy of woman and need to devalue her and overpower her has now been accepted by women. This acceptance, and the sense of worthlessness that it breeds, add to the powerlessness of women. The taboo feeds on itself:

> [given their dependency] . . . there is only one way for women to gain appreciation and be protected by men. They must do this by first concealing from men their genuine pleasure in their natural creativity. Then, unfortunately, they must conceal their pleasure from themselves and lay stress upon the other side of their role: the pain of labor connected with childbirth, the discomfort accompanying pregnancy, and the pain and discomfort of menstruation. Hence, they call the latter "the curse" or the "cramps," etc.[47]

If women focus on the "curse" rather than the pleasures associated with menstruation in order to placate men who have economic power (which we can easily admit) or the power to threaten us with rape (which is more difficult to admit as a psychic reality, although it is obviously a pragmatic one), the taboo of menstruation takes on many dimensions.

The taboo is tied to the needs of men but not to the inalienable rights of men. It has persisted for many thousands of years and in many different cultures because men have had the power to continue their domination of women. Freud would have us believe that men even own the deepest and most powerful psychic truths, but we have seen that this is the hypothesis of a man who was blind to the three-dimensional existence of woman.

The substance of woman includes her monthly bleeding and her monthly cycles. If women are to experience life fully, this reality must be reclaimed; in so doing, we may also expect to come into more direct contact with our fears of reprisal. That at least would be a prediction from the myth of the primal rape. If this myth is indeed the most accurate one, then the current battle for stronger rape laws and more conscientious prosecution of rapists may be seen as the foundation of woman's physical as well as her psychic freedom.

If woman is to reclaim her own image and her own body, she must be able to reduce the anxiety that rape will be her punishment. Woman must also reduce her dependency on man if she is to shake free from the taboo. While this is certainly difficult, it is at some level an approachable goal, free from the pulls of the psyche.

The diminution of the rape fear is more difficult because it is buried deep within us. It is also found to have a corollary in the sadistic inheritance of men. Perhaps we should not be altogether surprised, therefore, to find the rape statistics increasing as the freedom of women increases. Perhaps too we will not be altogether surprised to find that as women refuse to obey the constraints of the menstrual taboo, the fear of rape will also increase.

Should women take possession in full of their bodies, should women believe that menstruation and menopause are both natural and begin to partake of the pleasures inherent in both experiences, greater freedom will be felt—along with the substantial threats cited. The menstrual taboo, after all, is not a cultural oversight nor a habitual vestige of an outmoded life. It fills certain psychic and economic needs, it is alive, and it is flourishing. When the taboo is challenged, its beneficiaries also will be threatened—as will women who are not protected inside mental menstrual huts.

5

The Sexual Cycle

Menstrual blood flows from female genitalia. At the most basic anatomical level, sex, reproduction, and menstruation are related. Early education makes us believe that there is a hierarchy to the functions of the genital tract. Reproduction represents the highest aspect, and menstruation, the lowest, is in its service. Sexual activity is described as the mechanical method through which reproductive potential is realized. Once conception occurs, there is no further "need" for sexual activity, and there will be no more menstruation— for at least nine months.

The Puritanical heritage which provided the equation of reproduction and sexuality has been somewhat overturned. Conception and sexuality have been separated by the use of birth control devices; the nonmechanical, service-oriented approach to sexuality has been replaced by the liberation from the myth of vaginal orgasm and the myth of the sexually passive woman.

Many of us believe that the separation between sex and reproduction is now complete. We are free, at least potentially, to experience the full breadth of sexual feeling, unhampered by the old hierarchy of values which had diminished the sexual expectations of women. This belief exists only as long as we completely ignore the menstrual cycle; if we practice the menstrual taboo by burying the evidence of menstruation, we can believe that sexual freedom is a fact of modern-day life.

In the tradition against which we have rebelled, genitals were considered unclean. Touching them was verboten, and masturbation a moral transgression. These attitudes, of course, had their effect on the experience of menstruation:

I think my negative feelings [about menstruation] might in part come from my mother's attitude toward her children's genitals: When we would reach down to touch ourselves as all children do, she would slap our hands and tell us that the area was dirty. (s.s.)

We grew up and said, no more of this. The genitals are not dirty; they give us great pleasure. But our feelings about menstruation, the belief that *it* is dirty, did not disappear. It may be comforting to believe that the female genitalia have become a liberated zone, but as long as the menstrual taboo is in effect, this belief is an illusion.

If menstruation is unclean, so are woman's genitals. If menstruation is feared or considered "unattractive," then so are woman's sexual organs. To the extent that a woman believes in the attitudes surrounding the taboo, she will believe her sex and her sexuality are defiled. Sex and menstruation are most definitely connected.

The menstrual taboo has kept women from understanding this connection between sexuality and menstruation and from examining the relationship between the menstrual cycle and the sexual cycle. Indeed, in an attempt to reject the sexist argument that menstruation is a feminine impairment, we have too quickly reburied the very presence of cyclicity in all its forms.

Sexual Taboos

It seems preposterous to say that menstruation is a sexual experience. But it is.

The belief, of very ancient lineage, that coitus during menstruation led to the birth of monsters was formerly very widespread. . . . Ancient mythology attributed the deformity of Vulcan to the union of Jupiter with Juno during her menstrual period. The Talmud went further and assigned disorders of the mind, such as epilepsy, cretinism and insanity to the same cause. The belief is not wholly dead nowadays.[1]

Among the contemporary followers of Orthodox Judaism, sexual activity is prohibited for the duration of a woman's menstrual flow and for seven days thereafter. At the end of this entire period of time, a woman must go to the mikvah (ritual bath) and be cleansed. After the mikvah, sexual relations can be resumed.

The Brahmins of India are also forbidden to have intercourse during menstruation, but in their religion this lasts for only three days. At the end of three days, the woman must bathe, then until the next time of menstrual flow she is considered "clean."

Recently I had the opportunity to talk with women from Burma, Algeria, Venezuela, the Dominican Republic, Jamaica, Morocco, India, and Ethiopia. These women reported that in their home countries, as well as in the countries to which they have traveled (and they are all widely traveled) many, if not most, men and women practice abstinence during menstruation.

Not long ago a study of 960 Californian families showed that half the men and women abstained from intercourse during menstruation. Twenty-five percent of the women answering the menstrual questionnaire stated that they objected to intercourse during menstruation, while 41 percent said that male partners occasionally or frequently objected to sex at "that time of the month."

Karen Paige studied the effects of the menstrual taboo on female sexual behavior.[2] She reasoned that if women had less "mess, worry and fuss" with menstruation, they would be less likely to adhere to the taboo. She further hypothesized that women who had a lighter flow while using contraceptive pills would be less susceptible to the restrictions of the taboo than those whose flow had remained unchanged and was relatively heavy. To test her hypothesis she studied fifty-two women, all married and all of them using the pill. Fifty-five percent of the women in the study did not have sex during menstruation. When abstinence was correlated with amount of flow, however, she found that 62 percent of the women with normal flow did not have intercourse at menstruation, while only 35 percent of those with light flow abstained. In her opinion, women who have less menstrual "mess" have less allegiance to the taboo.

Among the respondents to the menstrual questionnaire, 196 (35 percent of all the women who answered) used the pill. Seventy-one women (12.7 percent of the total) used the IUD, and 75 women (13.4 percent of the total) the diaphragm. Since 75 percent of the women taking the pill reported a decrease in amount of flow and menstrual cramps, 73 percent of the IUD users reported heavier flow and cramping, and diaphragm users declared no method-related changes in menstrual experience, an analysis of these women's attitudes toward intercourse during menstruation might provide a useful comparison with Paige's study.

Thirty-five percent of pill users, 32 percent of IUD users, and 29 percent of those using the diaphragm reported that they preferred to abstain from intercourse while menstruating. More interesting still is an analysis of the reasons for their decision: of those on the pill, 19 percent said they objected to intercourse during menstruation because it was too messy; the same reason was given by 11 percent of the IUD users and by 16 percent of those using the diaphragm. Obviously the relationship between "mess, worry and fuss" and avoidance of intercourse is not so clear-cut. That there is some relationship, however, is indicated by another subcategory of response: 8.4 percent of women using the IUD said they avoided intercourse because the sheets got too bloody—a response made by only 2.5 percent of pill users and 1 percent of the diaphragm users. (Several women who use the diaphragm mentioned that it served the purpose of catching flow and also enabled them to keep menstruation to themselves literally and figuratively.)

Having noted that only 25 percent of the women responding to the questionnaire object to sex during menstruation but that 40 percent of their partners object, the question naturally arises: To what extent do women avoid intercourse because they fear their partners' negative response? Might the women in Paige's study who had less of the "mess" of menstruation appear to be relatively free from the taboo because their *partners*, and *not* the women, were less frequently repulsed by menstruation?

Although I cannot conclusively answer this question, I can point to the figures we found when we broke down the menstrual survey "partner objects" response category into subgroups according to the woman's method of contraception. We found that among partners of women taking the pill, 46 percent objected to sex during menstruation; 51 percent of partners of women using the IUD objected; while among partners of women using the diaphragm, objections occurred in only 40 percent of the cases.

The trend of these responses suggests that woman's choice of whether or not to have sex during menstruation is not strongly determined by the method of contraception she uses (although the methods do affect the amount of flow and pain). However, male preference about sex during menstruation appears to be determined in part at least by the method of contraception his partner uses and the amount of "mess" associated with the method.

To the extent that women are influenced by men's opinions, the male response to menstruation will affect the way women feel about sexual activity. Abstinence from sex during menstruation, whatever its component motives, supports and reinforces the menstrual taboo and confirms the belief that there is something wrong with menstruating women—something that makes sexual activity unappealing.

The presence of menstrual shame combined with sexual hibernation during flow corroborates the view that women are in fact less sexual than men. After all, if she cannot, or will not, have sex for a quarter of her life during the fertile years, she is "clearly" less sexual.

A study by Bardwick and Zweben on the psychological effects of contraceptive pill use illustrates this point. The investigators asked 150 college women: "Why do you make love?" These are some of the answers:

—I enjoy it to a certain extent. If I like the person, I have a desire to please rather than be pleased.

—I don't know. I think it's really necessary as a symbol of involvement.

—It's pleasurable, I guess. It's expected.

—It seems natural and because at this point it would harm the relationship not to.

—Besides the fact that it's a natural thing to do and we enjoy each other's company, want to feel united—and it's the first time I made a decision without someone helping me.[3]

The menstrual taboo, as demonstrated in the preceding chapter, has been one of the most successful methods devised to undermine the self-acceptance and confidence of women. It implies that there is something wrong with menstruation and, therefore, something faulty in our sexuality. By creating an atmosphere in which menstrual and sexual shame flourished, the groundwork was well prepared for woman to believe that her sexual activity was in the service of man and could not be an expression of *her* desires and feelings.

The taboo influences female experience because it is based on assumptions about how we ought to feel and how we ought to behave. Similarly, it influences the direction of research aimed at learning more about the connection between the menstrual cycle and sexuality.

As in any area of research, the focus and motivations of investigators vary; personal interests and prejudice must play a role in the formulation of projects. In this particular case, those who accept the taboo may find that some questions seem pressing while others never get asked. A set of basic assumptions colored by the taboo may result in research supporting it, even though the investigator is completely unaware of his or her personal prejudice.

Estrus and Menstruation

Does human sexuality represent a complete break with animal sexuality, or does the female of our species, like the members of other mammalian species, experience a period of heat? The answer to this question not only provides us with information about human sexuality; it also sheds light on the relationship between sex and the menstrual cycle. However, its very phrasing may lead to problems.

For some, the question is based on the assumption that sexual activity *must* be found to peak at the point of ovulation. This, of course, is the same as saying that sex must be related to conception. Certain investigators assume that the male of our species experiences a sexual drive which is not specifically related to reproduction, while the woman, if not quite labeled the servant of man, must be the servant of the species.

In most mammalian species, females go into heat (*estrus*), which is a convergence of internal and external events. Internally, ovulation is imminent; externally, the female engages in courtship, selects a mate, and copulates. Estrus is the only time when the female displays an active interest in sexual activity and when she is receptive to the advances of males. During periods in which she is not in heat, most, if not all, sexual forays on the part of males are rebuffed. And estrus is the *only* time she ovulates. The reproductive cycle is her sexual cycle.* If conception does not result from the sexual activity during estrus, the built-up lining of the uterus is reabsorbed, and the cycle is completed. In some species the next period of heat occurs within a short space of time (gerbils and rabbits come immediately to mind), while in other species it takes a seasonal course (bitches, for example, go into heat in the spring and fall).

---

* Although in these species copulation is always tied to ovulation, the sequence of events varies. In cats and rabbits, for example, estrus behavior begins, copulation occurs, and ovulation results from the stimulation of copulation. In bitches, ovulation occurs, and then copulation follows. With bitches, the staining seen during estrus is commonly likened to menstrual flow—it is not. Some women experience mid-cycle staining as a result of high levels of estrogen. This is very similar to the staining seen in bitches. It is breakthrough bleeding, not the shedding of the endometrium.

In the animal world, only three species have menstrual (rather than estrus) cycles: apes, Old World monkeys (of which the rhesus is an example), and humans. The reproductive cycle is approximately one month long and ovulation occurs, on the average, during mid-cycle. If conception does not occur during this cycle, the uterine lining is shed and expelled along with menstrual blood.*

Menstrual flow is not the only difference between the species that exhibit estrus and those that have menstrual cycles. In the menstruating primates, sexual behavior occurs throughout the reproductive cycle; it is not limited to the time of ovulation. Within this context it would appear that sexual behavior has become independent of reproductive potential. In other respects, of course, the menstrual and reproductive cycles are similar.

> It is important to realize that there is no essential physiological difference between heat or estrus cycles and menstrual cycles. The only new elements introduced by menstrual cycles are caused by a shifting of hormonal action and consist of (a) interestrus or continuous sexuality of a greater or lesser degree; and (b) the uterine build-up in preparation for a possible pregnancy so great that [it] . . . cannot be reabsorbed whether or not the embryo implants; it must be shed.[4]

Sherfey is surely correct here; yet the differences between estrus and non-estrus species are far greater than the physiological differences in reproductive actions. Certainly in the human being, sex is altogether independent of reproduction in many respects. Not only is there continuous sexual intercourse, but continuous sexuality which precedes the introduction of menstrual cycles and continues long after menstruation has finally ceased. For the human female alone, among mammalian species, sexuality is present from birth to death.†

As a menstruating species we are free from the constraint of sexual behavior which is completely determined by the time of ovulation. And, except where the taboo constraints are observed, we are free to

---

* Although sex and reproduction are separated in subhuman primate species, there remains a period of heightened sexual activity during the mid-cycle (ovulatory) phase. In the rhesus, for example, this is stimulated through vaginal production of an acidic secretion that acts as a sexual excitant for males. The very same vaginal secretion is manufactured in the human vagina. However, among some male members of our species vaginal odor is considered something less than sexually stimulating.

† There is not enough information available to make any statements about the nature of the clitoral response in subhuman primates, but among humans many have observed that from very early in development, females enjoy the sexual sensations this organ receives and transmits. Masters and Johnson have demonstrated that, as long as health permits, women can enjoy the pleasures of orgasm for the entire life span.

be receptive to sexual feeling throughout the menstrual cycle. Further, as human females, sexual feeling and its gratification are available throughout our life span. The independence of the sexual and reproductive cycles would appear to be complete.

While this analysis of the independence of sex and reproduction is true, it is not the entire story. During her menstruating years, a woman's sexual desire reflects the changes in hormone levels that control the menstrual cycle. There are, in fact, particular peaks of sexual interest which correspond to segments of the menstrual cycle. Woman's sexuality is not rigidly bound to reproduction, but it is *influenced* by changes in the reproductive (menstrual) cycle.*

Cycle of Sexual Arousal

In the 1930s, Benedek and Rubenstein[5] studied the relationship of the variation in sex hormone cyclicity and that of sexual desire. This work, which is now considered classic, is based on a physiological and psychological analysis of fifteen women who were in psychoanalytic treatment with Benedek. The time of cycle for each subject was established by hormone analysis, which showed when a woman was pre-ovulatory, ovulatory, and post-ovulatory. Records were kept of times of menstruation; 152 cycles were observed.

Benedek, a psychoanalyst and a follower of Freudian theory, saw these women throughout their cycles, since they were in treatment with her. In this way she had access to their reported thoughts and feelings at all times of the menstrual cycle. Furthermore, she analyzed their dreams and fantasies in an attempt to uncover unconscious sexual feelings. The results of their statements and her analysis were then correlated with the information about the stage of each cycle.

The women in this study said that the time they felt the greatest amount of sexual desire was near (or during) the time of menstrual flow. However, when she analyzed their dreams and fantasies and correlated them with the time of the cycle, Benedek concluded that

---

* Crawfurd reported that Captain Cook observed that among Eskimo women "not more than 10 percent . . . menstruated during the long winter months," and as though heightened desire were correlated to less frequent menstruation, a sexual season of great intensity set in at the first reappearance of the sun, and "little else was thought of for some time afterwards." This account of a seasonal heat for Eskimo women might be better understood as a function of the weight or fat loss during the long and less abundant winter and the return of menstruation when enough calories are supplied. It is an interesting observation also because it suggests that during the menstruating years, amenorrhea may imply a loss of sexual interest.

while women reported greatest sexual feeling around menstruation, they were actually most sexual at mid-cycle (the time of ovulation).

She based her conclusion on the kinds of sexual feelings expressed directly by the women and the kinds of feeling found in their dreams and fantasies. According to Benedek, the women felt most "loving" and "receptive" at the time of ovulation. In her view, this represents the highest form of female sexual expression. She states:

> The emotional cycle is always parallel to and dependent upon the gonadal cycle. In the evolution of the sexual cycle [for her, synonymous with menstrual cycle] woman reaches the highest level of psychosexual integration of which she is capable at about the time of ovulation when her physiological preparedness corresponds with her emotional preparedness for conception.[6]

She goes on to say that the reported high point of sexual feeling around the time of flow is really an expression of a lesser (lower) form of sexuality; these feelings represent an "impatient demand" for sex, and this period is filled with "extroverted activity and urgency." The qualities of urgency, demand, and extroversion present in female sexuality around the time of menstruation lead Benedek to conclude that this period of sexuality is more "masculine" in character. "Loving tenderness" combined with sexual feeling are evidently the proper, feminine forms of sexuality.

Surely, this conclusion is laden with value judgments we would be reluctant to accept. Why should we agree that receptivity is of higher value than extroverted activity? It is not higher or lower, but rather another dimension of female sexuality. To place a value judgment on types of sexual feeling and to call those around the time of ovulation "better" reflects the prejudices of an investigator who has started out with a view of what the female ought to be and assumes that when women are conforming to this vision, they are at the highest level of psychosexual development.

A woman struggling to learn about herself from the inside out has a rough time working through this study. Feelings are labeled better or worse as they fit into a researcher's narrow view of femininity—a view which also happens to be the stereotypical role of women.

The value judgments in this study are, of course, related to the menstrual taboo, and particularly to Freud's analysis of the woman question. Benedek adds substance to Freud's theory when she says that menstrually related sexual feelings in women are masculine rather than feminine. What is an acceptable feeling in a man becomes unacceptable in a woman, and furthermore is altered in a woman's body. The sexually aggressive man is being himself, as it were, while the extroverted and active woman is demonstrating a low level of psychosexual integration. In this impaired state she might represent a danger to man, as Freud suggested.

If the value judgments are ignored, however, several interesting facts emerge from the Benedek and Rubenstein study. It shows that women experience different sorts of sexual feelings and that there are several peaks of sexual interest. There is one peak around the time of ovulation and another near or during menstruation. Since the ovulatory peak is tied to a "loving" feeling, it can be perceived, expressed, and satisfied easily (at least in theory) in nonsexual ways, while the peak around menstruation is clearly sexual. Perhaps this, in part, explains why women report menstrual sexuality as the predominant experience of intensified sexual interest.

Kinsey and his colleagues[7] also sought to determine the time of cycle during which self-perceived sexual feeling was greatest. To do this they first asked women to relate the time of cycle when vaginal secretion was most profuse.*

Kinsey reports that among the 5,793 adult women in his study, those who had had sexual intercourse reported monthly variation of vaginal secretion. Sixty-nine percent experienced the most profuse secretion from one to four days before the onset of menstrual flow; 10 percent said it was greatest during flow; while 11 percent noticed the greatest secretion at mid-cycle.

Kinsey did a double check on these responses by asking these women when they felt most sexually aroused. The responses to this question directly paralleled those to the query about secretion. The vast majority of women felt most sexually aroused just before the onset of menstruation.

Women responding to the questionnaire I prepared also expressed the time of maximum sexual arousal to be near or during menstruation. Forty-five percent stated their peak was just before, during, or just after menstruation; only 6 percent said mid-cycle, and 35 percent that they experienced no cyclic alteration in sexual feeling.†

* As reviewed earlier (in chapter 2), vaginal secretion (of a nonpathologic sort) is greatest when sexual excitement is at its height. Kinsey reasoned, the more lubrication, the higher the level of excitement.
† It has been suggested that women might feel most sexual around the time of menstruation because they are not worried about becoming pregnant at this time. This assumes that women know when they are most likely to ovulate—an assumption not backed up by questioning. In my survey, for example, while

Udry and Morris[8] compared data from two already completed studies to investigate the relationship between the menstrual cycle and woman's sexual activity. Is the peak of activity really at menstruation at all? Perhaps, they might have pondered, women feel most sexual at mid-cycle, and by studying the incidence of intercourse and orgasm—not self-reported feelings—this could be proved. Their study pooled the reports of 90 women. The women were divided into three groups: single women (thirteen); married, working-class women (forty); and married, middle-class women (thirty-seven). Each of the working women had been asked to record frequency of sexual intercourse and orgasm and report the figures each day. The fifty other women kept a frequency record but submitted it to a researcher at the end of one year. The women were not asked to report on their sexual feelings or those of their partners.

In analyzing their results, the researchers report the existence of three sexual peaks experienced by the women in the study; one at mid-cycle, one just before, and one just after menstruation. The highest peak (representing greatest frequency of intercourse and orgasm) occurred at mid-cycle.

This study is as interesting for what it doesn't say as for what it does. While it corroborates some of the suggestions of the Benedek and Rubenstein investigation (that there is a peak of sexuality at the time of ovulation), it also includes some of the same assumptions.

Earlier in this chapter I included a sample of some of the reasons why women engage in sexual activity. Missing from that list was any mention of their own sexual feeling, but most definitely included were many mentions of the sexual feelings or supposed needs of their partners. Certainly the study done by Udry and Morris would have been more enlightening had they asked women to report on the presence or absence of sexual interest and the presence or absence of sexual interest on the part of their mates.

It is possible, for example, that the mid-cycle increase in receptivity demonstrated by the Benedek and Rubenstein study might have a definite effect on sexual activity because of the manner in which the male partner perceives the woman. The mid-cycle peak might reflect a higher frequency of intercourse (as Udry and Morris found) because men respond to the quality of receptivity in women, while the lower peaks around the time of menstruation might reflect men's disinterest in or dislike for more "extrovertedly active" partners. Had

---

45% of the women experienced maximum arousal co-incident with menstruation, only 20% knew the timing of ovulation.

the investigators asked for a record of which partner initiated sexual activity, as well as the frequency with which women initiated such activity and were met with disinterest, the study would have been that much more precise. In studies of sexual activity between men and women, it is essential to have access to information about the feelings and attitudes of *both* sexes. There is every reason to believe that male attitudes toward the quality of female sexuality have a profound influence on the shared experience. The study never attempts to answer why intercourse and orgasm are at their highest point during mid-cycle.

Kinsey found that women who may only masturbate once in each cycle do so in the few days before menstruation. Why is self-initiated orgasmic activity related to menstruation but shared activity most common at mid-cycle?

So far it has been shown that the peaks of female sexual feeling fall around the time of flow and at mid-cycle. Are there any low points of sexual interest among female humans, in relation to the menstrual cycle? Well, no one has spent any time looking. In this respect, I am also at fault, for I didn't ask this on my questionnaire. However, it is my experience that, for the women with whom I am well acquainted, the premenstrual week which culminates in heightened sexuality is preceded by a day or two of almost complete absence of sexual feeling—a sort of temporary anesthesia. Only further investigation will show how common this is.

During her menstruation years, a woman experiences a sexual cycle that parallels her menstrual cycle. For many women this means an increase of sexual desire near the time of ovulation and for most women a noticeable increase in sexual feeling around the time of menstrual flow. These facts of female life have been obscured by the menstrual taboo, and the results of the facts have promoted a good deal of sexual confusion and some amount of sexual frustration.

Women who believe it is "wrong" to have sexual intercourse during menstruation suffer in two ways: they experience a recurring period in which they think poorly of themselves, and, because of the generally common increase in sexual feeling, they are also likely to experience increased sexual frustration.

Women who are interested in sexual activity during menstruation but who have partners who believe this is "wrong" suffer from frustration perhaps, and may certainly suffer some amount of anger.

I have no objection, but I have been afraid to mention intercourse while menstruating for fear of being rejected by a partner. I have been afraid of discussing it. (C.M.S.-V.)

I think what really bothers me is the fact that my lover refrains from oral sex at this time. His semen excites me. I swallow it and rub it on my face and breasts. . . . I want as much understanding and love for my body. (A.C.)

This is one of the topics I feel most emphatic about. I recognize why, for example, men might be disgusted by making love with me while I am menstruating—intellectually. Emotionally, I feel strongly, as a woman, that he should be able to accept my body, my being, at all times of the month. That I accept into my body his discharge of semen and that my body is not "unclean" while I am menstruating. Also, I become quite easily sexually aroused at this time and do not feel that I should have to inhibit my activity. (S.S.)

It is reasonable to expect that when women become aware of the menstrual taboo and that rejection and distaste are not "natural" responses to menstruation but manifestations of the particular psychic structure of men, these male reactions will not be as readily accepted.

It is, of course, equally possible that awareness of the taboo and its implications may not change women's behavior. If the underlying taboo is understood and a woman *chooses* to accept it, we may presume the feeling she has will be different from what blind acceptance now dictates. Abstinence from intercourse while menstruating, for example, need not necessarily reflect negative assumptions about woman's role; it may be a response to some positive feelings about one's self and one's mate.

My sexual life centers a great deal around my period. My husband's and my sexual activity is directly related to the menstrual period. In ways, there are special advantages to the "period." It gives husband and wife a "rest" from each other—they enjoy each other in other ways. One's sexual experience and marriage get dull and you tend to take your spouse for granted.

The "Mikvah Experience" is not as fantastic as it seems though. It's difficult to be separate from your husband for twelve days (five days period—seven days afterward) but the advantages of keeping . . . the Laws of Family Life, far outweigh the disadvantages. (S.N.R.)

For some women, knowing when the probable peaks of sexual desire will come has a distinct practical advantage. Among women who have difficulty in reaching orgasm, this kind of knowledge might be helpful. Masters and Johnson have shown that in the luteal phase of the cycle, and especially near the time of menstruation, women most easily come to the plateau level of sexual excitement. This might be the best time to concentrate on orgasm.

We are accustomed to hearing that menstruation and menopause affect a woman's behavior. The changes described are always dreadful and debilitating—and they are harped upon by sexist men. Small wonder that we resist any implication that there is any behavioral aspect to either cycle of life. However, in the struggle to end the male definition of women, we do not have to blot out entire areas of our experience. We have already seen that there is a relationship between cyclicity and woman's sexual feeling. There also may be ways in which our behavior is influenced by the changes occurring during the cycles of menstruation. Harding cites an intriguing example:

> In her emotional life it seems that a woman's ability to respond to the opportunities life brings her depends very largely on her moon-phase [time of cycle] and this seems to be true in other realms as well. If the moment of the moon is favorable, her love can well up and respond to the man who attracts her, but if it happens to be an unfavorable moment, she remains cold and unresponsive, even though she may want to respond.
>
> I remember hearing the story of an abortive love affair whose miscarriage seemed to be largely due to this uncontrollable factor. A man and woman met and were much attracted to each other. Circumstances threw them together for about a week on two occasions. Then they each returned to their homes in different towns but they arranged, however, to meet again, for it so happened that his business took him to her town from time to time. From then on . . . fate was against them. For each time that he came, she was in an off phase and the incipient relationship gradually faded out. Such an outcome might just be called hard luck, or it could be taken more seriously.
>
> If her rhythmic changes were accepted by the woman as inherent in the nature of things, she might say with the ancients that the goddess, Ishtar, the moon, had gone to the land of No-Return, and so men and women could not love, they could only wait for her to come back.[9]

Ishtar . . . Could I invoke her name? Certainly to do so is to acknowledge the real existence of internal changes of feeling and to acknowledge, as well, certain limitations of the "mind." In the situation Harding (a Jungian analyst) described, I could be attracted to someone during the low point of my cycle, but my body and my emotions would temporarily not correspond.

To allude to Ishtar, in the context of Harding's description, is to stress the importance of our feelings as sexual beings. It also suggests that when the woman is not feeling sexual (and Ishtar is in the land of No-Return) the female experience of sexuality affects men sexually and emotionally, which presupposes respect for female sexuality—respect felt by women and men. All this considered, yes, I could call Ishtar's name.

Respect for female sexuality includes all the manifestations of our sexuality and cannot be limited by arbitrary timetables. The notion that women become sexual at menarche and stop being sexual at menopause is an adjunct of the menstrual taboo and has little to do with observed fact. The taboo, after all, is based on the premise that menstruating women are dangerous. Menstrual blood, therefore, contains an element capable of enormous power. It is a sexual element, but one that is most often believed to be destructive.

We all know that women are quite capable of turning the limitations of relative powerlessness into an advantage by playing upon the male belief that we possess secret and magical powers. This, too, applies to the male beliefs about menstruation:

> Menstrual fluid has always been reckoned to possess a powerful influence over the affections of men, and had held pride of place as an ingredient of the love-charms administered by girls to would-be lovers. In modern Germany, girls have administered drops of menstrual blood in coffee to their sweethearts to make sure of retaining their affections —a characteristic display of "frightfulness."[10]

Menstrual blood might be considered an aphrodisiac or it might be used by women in quite an opposite way. Traditionally, women have used their "headache" or curse as an excuse for avoiding sexual intercourse even when they are not menstruating. Although many women balk at the prohibition on sexual intercourse during menstruation, there are others who revive it by choice.

While it is possible to capitalize on the menstrual taboo, women are playing with volatile material when they choose to do so. The taboo, after all, is based on the belief that women are sexually dangerous for a quarter of each month. The three quarters of a month which remains is a time when woman is considered sexually desirable. In fact, her desirability is *enhanced* by the dangerous time of menstruation. When menstruation finally ends the taboo is no longer applied to woman. In men's eyes, her sexuality, no longer heightened by the presence of potentially dangerous menstruation, diminishes. Indeed, many men believe that menopausal and postmenopausal women are no longer sexually interesting or interested in a sexual life. Women who play upon the taboo, who reinforce it by their behavior, are reinforcing the association of menstruation with female sexuality and may be perpetuating the belief that female sexuality ends when menstruation ends.

A relationship between sexual feeling and the cycles of menstruation does exist and a greater awareness of the nature of this relationship may influence sexual activity. During the menstruating years, a sexual cycle parallels the menstrual cycle—peaks of sexual interest and heightened sexual responsiveness occur at both the peak of estrogen output and at the points of lowest estrogen production. The pattern of sexual feeling is affected by the existing levels of estrogen, but the existence of sexual feeling and responsiveness is not deter-mined by the presence of particular levels of this sex hormone.

Unlike the females of other mammalian species, the human female's sexual activity is not shaped by the physiological capability for conception. While the patterning of our sexual feelings is influenced by sex hormone levels during the years of menstruation and fertility, we are sexual long before fertility is initiated and long after it has ceased. Neither surgical removal of the ovaries nor the natural cessation of ovarian hormone production and egg extrusion generally has any effect on the intensity of female sexual interest or responsiveness.

We are the species in which sexual behavior is furthest removed from hormonal control. We are also the species that has demonstrated the greatest facility for conjuring up emotional constraints that are fully as limiting and confining as any physiological constraint might be.

6

Witch Doctors

Members of a tribe seek out their shaman or witch doctor when they are sick or believe they've been possessed by an evil spirit. He is the diagnostician and healer. Through techniques learned during years of apprenticeship he knows how to communicate with the spirit world, and this communication brings him to the source of an individual's physical or emotional problem. Once the source of the sickness has been divined, the shaman prescribes the appropriate medicine or tells the sufferer what actions must be performed to bring about cure. He may have learned that the problem stems from an infringement of spiritual law so extreme that the patient cannot be saved—at least by his ministrations. In such a case the patient may die or be banished from the community.

The shaman, because of his training, knowledge, and role, conserves the values of his society. He works to maintain the beliefs which give his culture shape and reinforces the power of the spirits who guide his people. The shaman cures by showing those who have strayed the way back onto the path of righteousness—unless, of course, they have strayed too far.

Psychoanalysts have been called the shamans of contemporary Western culture. Lévi-Strauss has elaborated this thesis in "The Sorcerer and His Magic."[1] The shaman uses his dreams, fantasies, and aberrations (brought about through trance or taking drugs) and the analyst uses the dreams, fantasies, and aberrations of his patients to learn the true nature of a problem.

The shaman takes his guidance from the spirit world, the medicine man from lore passed down the line of succession; the analyst uses the foundations given by analytic theory (the relation of this theory to the menstrual taboo was discussed in chapter 4). Each is privy to specialized information unknown to those who are not initiated. Like the shaman, analysts are essentially conservative figures, although they do not always like this description.

Female diviner at Nokong, Africa

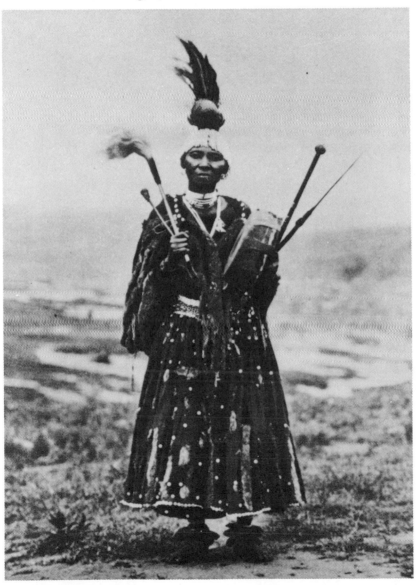

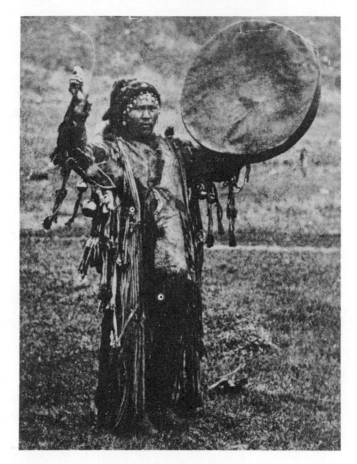

Medicine man of the Altai Mountains of Siberia

An analyst might prefer to say that he represents the forces of progress because his professed goal is to free a patient from the tyranny of unresolved internal conflicts. Not every analyst is completely guided by Freudian theory and certainly we are living in a time where the number of totally nonanalytic therapies is growing at a geometric rate.* However, analytic theory based on patriarchy and the unquestioned values of patriarchy has made its way into popular culture and affected the way many of us appraise one another and think about our problems. Theory is available in some form to most of us, but first-hand knowledge of its practical application is neither widely available nor universally dispersed.

* In 1974, a student of this subject reported the existence of sixty-five different types of therapy in San Francisco alone.

The analyst is not the Western equivalent of the shaman—he or she is simply not available to enough members of our tribe to qualify for this status. For women in modern-day America, however, another kind of shaman is consulted once or twice a year—even when no specific problem exists. In this culture, the gynecologist functions as witch doctor. The manner in which he views, diagnoses, and treats his patients' problems (especially those of menstruation and meno-pause) almost always reflects the conservative stance of his caste.

The Gynecologist as Shaman

The gynecologist has taken upon himself the role of diviner. He assesses the quality of normal female behavior—normal not only in the biological sense but in a social sense as well. By his own declarations he has specialized knowledge of a woman's body, her real spiritual potential, and the true nature of her unconscious mind.

If a gynecologist is conscientious, he will do a complete and careful physical workup before making his diagnosis. Should he find an organic problem (a tumor or polyp, for example), the woman with a menstrual or menopausal problem is treated like a medical "case." However, if he finds no pathological tissue, the woman is assumed to have a spiritual problem for which divine guidance is needed in order to make a diagnosis. Where does divine guidance lead him? Says Kroger:

> Menstruation is the "badge of femininity." Whether it is worn in misery, pain or pride depends on a woman's attitude toward herself as a female, and her biologic destiny—marriage and motherhood.[2]

and Kaufman:

> But how does woman accept middle age? Not with open arms but with clenched fists. . . . She is concerned with each added year, each added pound, each new gray hair. She worries that she is becoming less attractive to her husband. If he is busier than ever and seems less attentive, she interprets this as rejection. Her children may have grown to the point of no longer needing her. She may find it difficult to keep a job or get a new one. If she is single, she sees her chances of marriage slipping away with each passing year. If on the other hand, she had been happily married and is now widowed, she must adjust to an irreplaceable loss.
>
> In short, she sees loneliness ahead. . . . She begins taking a sleeping pill at night, and tranquilizers during the day. Perhaps a couple of

extra drinks now and then. She may become moody and depressed, suffer from fatigue. . . .

And it is in this setting that menopause arrives. It couldn't be at a worse time.[3]

The gynecologist has assumed leadership as the enforcer of the menstrual taboo and its adjunct, the mythic menopause. From menarche through menopause, it is this physician/shaman who interprets the meaning of her physical problems and points to the woman's failure to obey the rules of femininity as the cause of the problem—rules implicit in the taboo. He shows her the cure (in the form of social readjustment) and tells her she must more rigorously conform to the female role—a role *he* defines.

If a woman is not married, marriage will "cure" her. If she is already married, children will cure her. If she is already married and mothering, then more diligent performance of these roles will cure her. If she is not a mother and is in menopause, she must accept this position as best she can in order to effect a partial cure.

Doctors' remedies: "Wait until you grow up and have a baby, then things will work out." At thirteen I wasn't too excited by that answer. . . . I continued to receive this answer until my late teens when I started answering the doctor more bluntly. (ANON.)

Most of the "old wives' tales" came from doctors! . . . I have seen many doctors for menstrual cramps. . . . Most . . . use a sappy "think positive" approach—"those cramps are all in your head." (A.M.)

In his capacity as physician/shaman, the gynecologist has taken control of both the medical and spiritual guidance of the lives of many women.* In his role as witch doctor, the gynecologist uses his medical-school training but combines it, in a peculiar admixture, with a watered-down version of psychoanalytic theory.

Gynecologists are not tortured with doubts about the finer points of analytic theory, nor are they concerned with what has been left unexplored in the psychology of women. They appear to be satisfied

---

* In every women's health course, at every women's meeting, most women report that they regularly see a gynecologist but not a family doctor or internist. Once or twice a year, at least, a woman must see a physician for a Pap smear, birth control, vaginal infections, and other routine female health concerns regardless of whether or not she is in overall good health. Like men of the same age, many women do not need or cannot afford regular consultations with an internist unless they get sick. But women are learning that an internist can perform the same standard tests and examinations as a gynecologist and that internists, lacking the cultural status, do not assume the role of the shaman.

that enough is known—and "enough" seems to mean the most simple-minded translation of theory into medical practice.

Gynecology textbooks are riddled with statements about the psychological or sociological roots of menstrual and menopausal distress.[4] Despite feelings of vulnerability and menstrual shame, women have repeatedly attempted to tell their physicians that the problems are not in their heads but in their bodies. The doctor, convinced his theory is the right one, pays little attention to what his patients have to say.

> There are no standing requirements either in the residencies or as part of the Specialty Board examinations for an ob-gyn to demonstrate any competence in any aspect of behavioral science, human development, psychology of women, or even psychology in general. Every woman should understand that what this means is just because a doctor is a certified ob-gyn doesn't mean that he is qualified or trained or prepared in any way to give advice or counsel . . . in any human-relations area of a woman's life.[5]

Women should understand and remember that gynecologists do not generally have any special training in psychology and, for the moment, seem content to osmose analytic theory and freely translate it into practice.

Almost every woman has had menstrual pain at some time in her life. Freudian analysts believe that menstruation is a sorrowful experience:

I was going to a psychoanalyst once, and I told him I didn't enjoy getting my period because I usually got a lot of cramps. He said the real reason for my dislike of menstruation was the fact that I wanted to be a boy and I hated to be reminded that I wasn't (D.M.M.)

Helene Deutsch says that:

> Menstrual pains constitute another complication of the normal course of development. This manifestation . . . has many causes, of which some are general and some individual. Most authors who have studied the psychological processes accompanying such pains connect them with birth fantasies.[6]

Deutsch goes on to discuss menstrual pain and finds it impossible, even using analytic techniques, to be sure whether a woman's pains stem from such birth fantasies or whether in fact the fantasies emerge out of the pain. This is a dilemma, both theoretical and practical, for a thoughtful analyst, but not for the more casual analyst or the psychologically casual gynecologist. To many gynecologists menstrual pain is the most decisive evidence that a woman has failed to accept the female role. This has led to a vicious cycle in which women suffer the most severe discomfort, go to a doctor for help, are told they are psychologically responsible for their pain, and leave the doctor's office in physical and mental agony. As the Lennanes put it:

> Dysmenorrhea, nausea of pregnancy, pain in labor, and infantile behavioral disturbances are conditions commonly considered to be caused or aggravated by psychogenic factors. Although such scientific evidence as exists clearly implicates organic causes, acceptance of a psychogenic origin has led to an irrational and ineffective approach to their management.[7]

Among the many possible problems associated with menstruation and menopause, dysmenorrhea is the only one to be re-evaluated. The admonitions of patients were not successful in shaking gynecologic convictions, but the Lennanes' paper, appearing in the prestigious *New England Journal of Medicine*, gave the stonewalling shamans a sizable jolt. They were being accused of mismanagement of a medical problem and irrationality in their persistence by peers; this could no longer be *completely* ignored.

A growing number of gynecologists now consider menstrual pain a physical problem and no longer immediately jump to the field of psychodiagnosis. However, the premise that menstrual and menopausal problems are more a product of the patient's mind than of her body still holds firm, although menstrual pain has been removed from the list of *a priori* proofs of instability.

Listen, doctors know so little. Some admit it, others pretend they know it all. . . . What bothers me are the [menstrual] depressions and having mentioned it casually to one doctor, I've decided not to mention it to others. Either they think dinner out with your husband is all that's needed, or I'm afraid of getting one who'll lock me up as a potential suicide. (B.T.)

Depression. . . . Sometimes it's virtually nonexistent and sometimes it's debilitating. . . . I haven't mentioned it to a doctor for a long time because when I did it was called a neurotic problem. (It's worse when taking the pill.) (J.C.)

Fifty to 75 percent of women experience one or more premenstrual symptoms. Eighty to 90 percent have at least one menopausal symptom. Depression is common to both premenstrual and menopausal syndromes. Because depression is clearly a mental experience, it fits perfectly into the gynecologist's framework, and he cites it as evidence of the lack of emotional adjustment in the menstrual or menopausal patient.

Menstrual or menopausal depression may, of course, be symptomatic of a psychological conflict. Gynecologists, however, do not often trouble themselves with the finer distinctions of psychodiagnosis; nor, unfortunately, do all psychiatrists.

> Menstrual depression has been related to a failure to conceive. . . . Menninger explains the syndrome as a woman's rejection of her femininity: "The envy of the male cannot be repressed and serves to direct her hostility in two directions: she resents the more favored and envied males while secretly trying to emulate them, and at the same time she hates and would deny her own femaleness."[8]

Menninger's vision of the etiology of menstrual depression is similar to Freud's explanation of the origins of the taboo on virginity found in some preliterate societies. Like Freud, he seems to be suggesting that menstruation is rightfully taboo because woman's rage and envy, naturally and inevitably unleashed when she has "failed" to conceive, are no longer controllable. The taboo is the natural outgrowth of the male response to the dangerous emotionality of women. The symptom of depression (or whatever symptom appears) is then cited as proof of woman's menstrual derangement. (In this framework depression is considered a salient symptom because it results when anger is turned inward.)

The drugstore psychoanalyst or the gynecologist/shaman might find this explanation of menstrual or menopausal depression satisfactory and use it in practice, but it stands as a convoluted and tyrannical solution to a medical puzzle.

Berry and McGuire conducted an experiment to study the relationship of menstrual symptoms to the acceptance of the sexual role.[9] This study was performed in 1972, and it is noteworthy that no one had conclusively demonstrated that sex role maladjustment caused premenstrual syndrome. (This is an experimental question which doctors have continued to ignore.)

In their study, Berry and McGuire tested one hundred women who were patients in a state mental hospital. These women were "in contact with reality" and were all between the ages of menarche and premenopause. After analyzing the data obtained, the researchers found that a significant number of women who experienced menstrual pain showed a low level of acceptance for the female role.

However, women with premenstrual tension (of which depression is a component) had a level of sex role acceptance that was in the normal range. Depression associated with menstruation, therefore, should not be considered proof of a woman's resistance to being female.

These investigators reasoned that people can more easily cope with tension than pain. The pairing of menstrual pain and low acceptance of being female would have a logical base. The relationship of menstrual pain and low sex role acceptance, they said, "is not a surprising finding since it would be logical to assume that most women would be unhappy with a role which required such discomfort for much of their lives."[10]

This conclusion, of course, is not news to the millions of women who have suffered from menstrual pain, but it is so symptomatic of gynecologic authoritarianism and tyranny that its logic is lost on them.

Sound medical and analytic practice would dictate that a medical problem, whatever its possible psychogenic origins, should always be studied by thorough physical examination and the necessary tests to arrive at a medical diagnosis. If a diagnosis cannot be confirmed, medical management of the possible physiological malfunction should be undertaken; and if conscientious medical methods do not succeed, the time may come to consider other methods of diagnosis and treatment. Premature psychogenic diagnoses have cost women thousands and thousands of dollars, years of frustration, and perpetuation of symptoms. It has caused thousands of other women, who do not seek the recommended analytic treatment or agree with gynecological psychoanalysis, to go through life with their physical symptoms intact and their sense of worth severely damaged.

In many cases, of course, where temporary internal or external stresses have led to a symptom of menstrual or menopausal distress, neither protracted medical testing nor psychological treatment are necessary.

Any form of stress, whether from pleasant or painful situations, may be responsible for menstrual irregularity, including bleeding irregularities and change of cycle length. Stress can provoke outbreaks of menopausal hot flushes or sleeplessness. A change in job, moving to a new house, taking a trip, or a new course of study can and frequently do affect menstrual and menopausal experience. Even anticipating one of these changes can result in a change of hormone production. These stresses are, of course, transient.

Severe and more prolonged stresses can obliterate cyclicity and greatly exacerbate the symptoms of menopause. For example, women living in combat zones, and those incarcerated in concentration camps, prisons, or mental institutions, may lose the menstrual cycle altogether.

Whether the initial cause is something as minor as taking a vacation or as traumatic as living in a war zone, the alterations in menstrual cyclicity or menopausal experience add stress of their own. In the more minor situation, of course, this can be coped with rather easily, although worry could be reduced or alleviated altogether by the simple knowledge that it is not mysterious or malign. In a traumatic situation the suppression of menstruation can be so upsetting that one's ability to cope goes beyond the breaking point.

In *Going Places,* a movie released in the United States in 1974, Jeanne Moreau plays a character who has just been freed from a lengthy stay in prison. She uses her very first contact with another woman (a waitress at a seaside restaurant) to talk about what prison has done to her and tells the startled waitress that in prison she had stopped menstruating. The waitress, taken aback by this "inappropriate" and certainly unsolicited confession, tells Moreau that she is sorry but also suggests that it is none of her business. Moreau, with great feeling, responds by saying that she simply wanted the other woman to understand what it really means for a woman to be in prison; in effect, she is saying that the loss of her womanhood (menstruation) was cruel and unusual punishment for the (unnamed) crime she committed.*

For some women the suppression of menstruation could be a blessing, but for others it could be the final deprivation in a life of deprivation. Between these extremes, the appearance of menstrual or menopausal symptoms or the disappearance of menstruation are

---

* Like the other women in this movie, the character played by Moreau is drawn from a male fantasy of the female. It is the male who has imagined that menstruation "means" female, and that its loss would naturally be sexually devastating. While women's attitudes toward menstruation vary, the *absolute* evaluation of femininity with menstruation must be seen as an outgrowth of the taboo. The fantasies on which the taboo is founded are elaborated later in the film when Moreau commits suicide (another act without apparent motive). She shoots a gun into her vagina and, in death, bleeds once again from her genitals. No doubt there are women who have completely internalized the male myth of femininity and who would prefer death to an "unfeminine" (nonmenstruating) life—though I've never heard of such a woman existing off screen. However, as was the case in the earlier confessional scene, this attitude reflects male fantasies and convictions wholly believed by a woman. This suicide scene was devastating because it so graphically and violently demonstrated one logical outcome of the life of a woman who is completely defined by men, and because (however limited its extent) we are all still defined by men.

likely to be sources of some anxiety and will only complicate the stresses already present. In these cases (and perhaps in those that appear to be more extreme) knowledge of the relation between stress and the fluctuations of the female sex hormones might be enough to end the chain reaction of anxiety. The problems of menstruation and menopause will, in the case of transient environmental or emotional stress, clear up by themselves. As Virginia Woolf puts it: "What is meant by "reality"? It would seem to be something very erratic, very undependable—now to be found in a dusty road, now in a scrap of newspaper in the street, now in a daffodil in the sun."[11] No one has a monopoly on reality, least of all the shaman/gynecologist. In most cases the woman herself is the best equipped to know if a menstrual change or menopausal flare-up is the likely result of a stressful situation and whether the stress is temporary or long-standing.

Female biochemistry is one reality, worry another, and unresolved psychic conflicts still another. Reality is also found in the structure of a culture which asserts that menstruating woman is a fearsome being and menopausal woman a sad, powerless creature. The reality defined by a man's world and promoted by gynecologists is filled with language that describes woman's envy of the penis, her weeping womb, and menstruation as the failure of conception but the badge of femininity. Not much is heard about the psychic response of men to the monthly bleeding of women, nor of their response to women who no longer have menstrual cycles. Man's projection onto woman of all that he fears and would rather not identify within himself appears to be complete; among that group of men who play at being shamans, it *is* complete.

Gynecologists, after all, are only members of the society along with every other man and woman. They have been raised in a culture where menstruating woman is taboo and menopausal woman a pathetic or unsexed creature who has simultaneously outlived the taboo and her usefulness. However, if this were completely true, gynecologists would, like the rest of us, be passive transmitters of the social code. But they are not; they actively enforce the taboo.

Roots of the Shaman's Power

The gynecologist is not just another member of the tribe. We may well wonder how he came to be the maker of magic and, considering the havoc he has created, how he is able to maintain his position. Lévi-

Strauss has described the conditions which must be met if the principles and actions of magic are to have effect. He says that three sets of conditions must exist:

> First, the sorcerer's belief in the effectiveness of his techniques; second, the patient's or victim's belief in the sorcerer's power; and, finally, the faith and expectations of the groups, which constantly act as a sort of gravitational field within which the relationship between sorcerer and bewitched is located and defined.[12]

The shaman believes that he is apart from the culture and in a transcendent state of communication with the gods; the gynecologist comes to this inflated self-image in several ways. First, he is a medical doctor, and physicians are trained to behave authoritatively whether or not they're sure of what they're doing. Their training is so thorough that by the time they become M.D.'s they believe their judgments are infallible. "The power of physicians in most Western societies . . . the imputation of competence and the false accordance to them of trust, has served to shield the knowledge and practices of the medical profession, including the quality of their research."[13]

Medical research, and especially research which might answer basic questions about menstruation and menopause, is impaired because the doctor is content with his magic and makes few demands on his science. While the shaman may enjoy his power, its practice is rarely pleasurable for his patient. Alice James (sister of Henry and William) articulates the patient's point of view with a voice both delicate and cutting:

> *September 27, 1890*
> . . . These doctors tell you that you will die, or *recover!* I have been at these alterations since I was nineteen and I am neither dead nor recovered—as I am now forty-two, there has surely been time for either process. I suppose one has a greater sense of intellectual degradation after an interview with a doctor than from any human experience. . . .[14]

The gynecologist is "more royal than the King." After a round or two with his authoritarian ways, his patient is very likely to shut up and let him think whatever he pleases. The Lennanes have pointed out that:

> The terms commonly used to describe the psychic difficulties—"neurotic" and/or "unfeminine"*—are, to the laity, simply derogatory, and

* In this case, gynecologists are in fact part of the lay population and hardly free from the value judgments that "neurosis" and "unfemininity" are derogatory expressions.

patients reluctant to be so classified may be unduly complaisant, uncritical, and "feminine" in their behavior, and reluctant to report symptoms or failure to respond to treatment.[15]

They have described the gynecological Catch-22. If a woman's menstrual or menopausal problem is diagnosed as "failure to be sufficiently feminine" and she tells the doctor that despite his ministrations the problem remains, she is being "unfeminine," which proves his diagnosis was right. If she keeps quiet, he can go on believing that

Le Toucher, *by J. P. Maygrier, 1822*

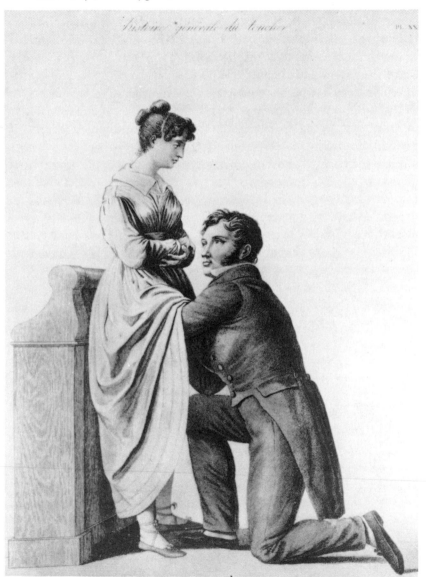

his diagnosis was correct from the beginning and his prescription a miracle drug. The patient continues to have the problem, but he is convinced it is cured. If she should try to speak up again, she is called aggressive and unfeminine; the more she talks, the more confirmed the diagnosis.

The shaman skillfully manipulates the themes of this vicious circle and thereby reinforces his position—the woman is always in the wrong and he alone can set her right. He alone can identify the source of her problem, which he finds almost always in transgressions of the taboo. Punishment rapidly follows, yet the penalty is cast in the light of help. If she will only listen, her problem will disappear. If she refuses to do so, her problems will continue, perhaps get worse, and the doctor will no longer take responsibility for her welfare.*

A woman's doctor might be expected to educate his patients about their bodies—but the shaman is not an educator, he is a diviner who mouths incantations about the sex role and has the power to identify those who have strayed from those who keep walking the straight path.

The majority of doctors have an elevated opinion of their worth and an undeveloped ability to respect their patients. The shaman/gynecologist plays upon the vulnerability of his patients with relative ease. He freely uses analytic concepts despite his utter lack of well-grounded education in psychology—and he believes what he is saying. The ease with which he assumes this role can be traced to the fact that 97 percent of gynecologists are male, while 100 percent of their patients are female.

If the magical system is to work, women (the object of the magic) must support it. Before a woman ever crosses the doorstep of the gynecologist's office she is imbued with shameful feelings about menstruation and menopause; she believes deep inside that menstruation is an unclean, damning pattern and that menopause is the end of her sexual identity.

In accepting the taboo, we accept a male vision of who and what women are. This also implies agreement with the male's view of himself—he is the more important and powerful and his opinions are worth more than ours, even when they are about ourselves. The gynecologist, a man, is telling women that the menstrual taboo must

---

* In the last few years, more and more women have begun challenging the authority of their gynecologists. As a result, more and more women are reporting instances in which these good doctors answer in ominous tones: "I will not be responsible for your health." To a woman who is worried about her health this response can hardly be considered professional, but it is the apt reply of a man with magical powers which "shall not be questioned."

be obeyed. We are likely to be somewhat vulnerable to his prescriptions.

The feelings that underlie the taboo are rarely experienced directly by men because they are successfully projected onto women. A man doesn't need to feel afraid, because *we are*. We are not afraid of ourselves—we are afraid of him. The gynecologist, for example, does not feel terror when he treats his patients. He may feel filled with understanding and wisdom. He believes that he will help each woman to find her true self and show her the way to become more feminine. And once this is accomplished, he feels, the patient will no longer suffer so terribly from the curse of menstruation and the ridiculous pain of menopause.

To the extent that we continue to believe even a fraction of the ideas contained in the taboo, we have a right to be frightened because if we are not properly feminine within its framework there is a great deal to lose. The anthropologist Ruth Benedict wrote a diary entry in which she outlined her vision of femininity:

> So much of the trouble is because I am a woman. To me it seems a terrible thing to be a woman. There is one crown which perhaps is worth it all—a great love, a quiet home, and children. We all know that this is all that is worthwhile, and yet we must peg away, showing off our wares on the market if we have money, or manufacturing careers for ourselves if we haven't. We have not the motive to prepare ourselves for a "life-work" of teaching, of social work—we know that we would lay it down with hallelujah, in the height of our success, to make a home for the right man.[16]

If woman's work is to prepare herself for this moment, then she believes in the male definition of her role. She is to love and care for a man and their children. If she is to get this love, obviously in his eyes she must be feminine. Enter the gynecologist/shaman.

A woman who believes herself liberated will take issue with this, or rather, she will say that it doesn't apply to *her*. The menstrual taboo with its definitions of femininity and the entire capitulation to male definition of the female isn't real for her. However, when the liberated woman finds herself at the shaman's office with her feet in the stirrups she understands his language very well. In some corner of our hearts we still harbor the myths of femininity, and in proportion to the intensity of this hidden belief, we are still vulnerable to his magic. The "free" woman may be less susceptible, but it is difficult to believe she is completely immune.

In Lévi-Strauss's formulation, the last component necessary for the maintenance of magic belief is the "faith and expectations of the group." The power given to the gynecologist, the conviction that menstruation is unclean, menopause ludicrous, and his collection of psychoanalytic concepts (penis envy or female genital rage as a prime mover in mental development)—all demonstrate the faith and expectations of our group.

Not long ago a friend told me a story about an experience in medical school. A physician was "presenting" a psychiatric patient for study. When he described her pre-hospital sexual activities he mentioned that, naturally she did not have sexual relations during menstruation. My friend went on to say that she could tell which of the men in the group had had sex with menstruating women just by looking at the expressions on their faces following this remark—half of them were smiling, the other half looked puzzled by the smiles. Not one of these present or future psychiatrists questioned the assumptions implicit in the remark, nor did any of them discuss the analytic theories which support the taboo. One might assume that although some of these students didn't obey one of the laws of taboo, by their silence they nonetheless subscribed to its underlying definitions.

Because the gynecologist/shaman is woman's doctor, he is the specialist in "female complaints and delicate condition." The male-centered society has every reason to support the shaman in his assumption of responsibility for women during "that time of the month" or "that time of life." After all, the menstruating woman is considered a source of a potentially destructive electrical charge which until menopause has passed is a constant threat. Within this context the shaman has the function of a lightning rod which safely deflects the danger. Women don't believe themselves possessed by an evil menstrual spirit but may nonetheless bow to those who detect this evil and to the profession whose job it is to render it neutral.

As the women's liberation movement of recent years began to expand, many women took a new look at the unbreakable commandment of femininity—Thou shalt defer. Not surprisingly, gynecologists, who for so long had told us how to be feminine, have come in for a great deal of abuse as a result.

> We can be angry . . . and we should be, but it is a mistake perhaps to look for confirmation from the doctor of our feelings and identity as women in the first place. That is where only a group of women, being honest with themselves and one another, can hope to sort it all out.[17]

Thousands of women have now participated in women's groups, and thousands more have learned about their bodies in women's health courses. For the majority of women who have shared these experiences, there is little doubt that women can help one another learn what it means to be a woman. Chesler considers that: "Up to a point, women's liberation was more therapeutic than either marriage or psychotherapy; it made women happier, angrier, more confident, more adventurous, more moral and it produced a wide range of behavioral changes."[18] Women have begun to question the tyranny of gynecologists and to express their anger. And women have also learned that there are instances when a menstrual or menopausal problem *is* an outgrowth of some psychological conflict. It is always tempting to deny that an emotional problem is at the core of a physical one—if one were easily able to identify a mental problem for what it is, the physical symptom would not have developed in the first place. Denial is even more tempting when gynecologists step in. When a woman considers the possibility of a psychological cause for a menstrual or menopausal problem, it seems like an invitation to the shaman to rush in and take charge of the proceedings.

In women's groups, it soon became obvious that most of the problems with menstruation and menopause result from physical malfunction or cultural pressures. The individual woman whose problems appear to be the result of personal, internal conflict can gain strength from the support of other women and can consider what she wants to do next. She may choose a form of psychological therapy and, through women's groups, get the names of therapists who do not perform the function of conserving patriarchy. Or she may make another kind of choice.

Pooling knowledge and sharing feelings are not going to solve all the problems of menstruation and menopause. This will not work for the individual woman in internal conflict, and it will not work for us as a sex. Sharing and learning are not going to make the magical world of the shaman disappear, any more than sharing can make the physical problems associated with menstruation and menopause disappear. And when a physical problem exists we may well need medical attention.

How are we to place ourselves in the care of men with a complacent and warped view of women? How are we going to successfully change the relationship between women and the gynecologist? Perhaps we could begin by following the path suggested by Virginia Woolf:

The pleasure of dominance is of course further complicated by the fact that it is still, in the educated class, closely allied with the pleasures of wealth, social and professional prestige. Its distinction from the comparatively simple pleasures—e.g., the pleasure of a country walk— is proved by the fear of ridicule which great psychologists, like Sophocles, detect in the dominator; who is also peculiarly susceptible according to the same authority either to ridicule or defiance on the part of the female sex. An essential element in this pleasure would seem to be derived not from the feeling itself, but from the reflection of other people's feelings, and it would follow that it can be influenced by a change in those feelings. Laughter as an antidote to dominance is perhaps indicated.[19]

7

Congratulations,
Today You Are
a Woman

During puberty girls change every day and sometimes, it seems, every minute. One day the girl is a child, the next an adult, the third a child again. She swings back and forth, leaping across huge intervals of time. Adults perceive a woman's body emerging from that of a girl and watch her as she tries on adult emotions and attitudes. We believe that we are standing at the sidelines, cheering her on, offering gentle guidance, and wish her the best.

The emergence of womanhood is observed by adults whose response is not limited to good will, however. Fear is buried within us and what appears beautiful at some moments is terrifying at others. A year or more after the process of puberty begins, the first menstrual flow appears. Menarche is the sign and symbol of womanhood. It is the index of female sexuality as well as the potential for reproduction.

These two predominant attitudes toward woman converge and are amplified at menarche, signaling the beginning of fertility—woman's greatest blessing. But menarche is also the result of completion of the first full menstrual cycle, a cycle which each month culminates in the flow of blood—and menstrual blood, said to be unclean, is a symbol of the dangerous contamination unleashed by female sexuality in its purest form.

Adults respond to menarche with a mixture of delight and embarrassment. They delight in the young woman's fertility (as long as she doesn't get pregnant), but her menstruation makes them uncomfortable. Shame is not acknowledged, of course; indeed, it is denied as completely as possible. We pretend that menarche is an important event in a girl's life because she has now become a fertile young woman, but we don't make too much of this day for fear that the ambiguity of our feelings would have to be acknowledged. In this way fears are shunted aside and the implications of menarche remain hidden—from adults as well as from young women.

Since 1830, menarche has advanced by four months in each decade. In 1830 the average age at menarche was seventeen; today, it is between twelve and thirteen.* The physical appearance of a young woman begins to change a year or even two years before menstruation. Young women are expected to act as girls until social convention establishes the appropriate time for entry to adulthood, but social convention has not kept pace with changes in biological maturity. A girl begins to look like a woman when she is ten or eleven; yet adults continue to expect her to remain a child until she is fifteen or sixteen. While social maturity has always followed closely behind physical maturity, our culture has tried to keep the two apart. Sexual puritanism lives on, and we continue to assert that it is improper for young women to behave as sexually matured beings until they are well into their adolescence. Adults point to the accelerated pace of modern-day life, as exemplified in such inventions as television, as the reason the young have been led astray—as though the cathode-ray tube might be responsible for the "precocious" development of young people. A higher standard of living and the better diet it offers has led to the earlier age of physical and social maturity; television had nothing whatever to do with it.

> The peasant girls of this landschard in general menstruate much later than the daughters of the townsfolk or the aristocracy, and seldom before their seventeenth, eighteenth or even twentieth years. . . . The townsfolk have usually borne several children before the peasant girls have yet menstruated. The cause seems to be that the inhabitants of the town consume more fat food and drink so their bodies become soft, weak and fat and come early to menstruation.[1]

The arrival of a critical weight, reflecting a critical ratio of fat to lean tissue, triggers the onset of menstruation. If young women were taught this, if they were not left alone to make up whatever explana-

---

* The present age at which the critical weight is attained reflects improvements in health care and nutrition. The critical weight has not changed appreciably in a century; what has changed is the age of arrival. As a result of higher standards of living, the age at menarche may soon stabilize not far below the present 12.9 years.

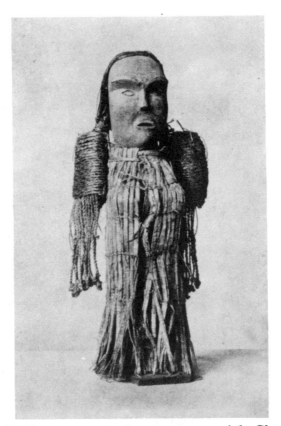

A doll dressed in the costume worn by young women of the Clayoquat Indian tribe in British Columbia at the time of their first menstrual flow

tions suited their imaginations and fears, they would be spared a lot of confusion and unhappiness. But young women in our culture are not taught about critical weight or many other aspects of menstrual experiences because adults close their eyes and ears to the phenomenon of menstruation.

Rites of Passage

In many cultures where menstruation is taboo, menarche is the occasion for special ceremony. While the taboo, whatever its form, will have a negative influence on the young woman's concept of female identity, the ritual of welcoming her to her new status pro-

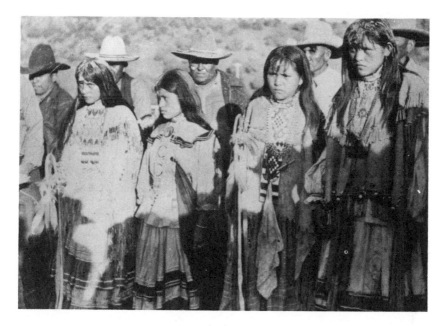

Young Apache women about to begin the ceremony that marks the onset of menstruation. Behind each girl is the medicine man who will guide her through the ritual.

vides her with some positive experience she can include in her conception of womanly identity. Furthermore, such rituals give an external form to the internal changes of puberty and adolescence. This structure helps a young woman learn that the biological and social changes she is experiencing are part of the known world and, to some extent at least, an acceptable part of that world. In this way she is helped to develop an integrated sense of her identity rather than the fragmented identity that is the inheritance of women in Western culture. Margaret Mead describes the ritual performed among the members of the Arapesh people, members of a preliterate society:

> A girl's first menstruation and the accompanying ceremonial take place in . . . her husband's home. But her brothers must play a part in it and they are sent for; failing brothers, cousins will come. Her brothers build her a menstrual hut, which is stronger and better-constructed than are the menstrual huts of older women. . . . The girl is cautioned to sit with her legs crossed. Her woven arm and leg bands, her earrings, her old lime gourd and lime spatula are taken from her. . . . If these are fairly new they are given away; if they are old they are cut off and destroyed. There is no feeling that they themselves are

contaminated, but only the desire to cut the girl's connection with her past.

The girl is attended by older women who are her own relatives or relatives of her husband. They rub her all over with stinging nettles. They tell her to roll one of the large nettle-leaves into a tube and thrust it into her vulva: this will ensure her breasts growing large and strong. The girl eats no food, nor does she drink water. On the third day, she comes out of the hut and stands against a tree while her mother's brother makes the decorative cuts upon her shoulders and buttocks. This is done so gently, with neither earth nor lime rubbed in —the usual New Guinea method for making scarification marks permanent—that it is only possible to find the scars during the next three or four years.[2]

In the south of India and in Ceylon, present-day members of the Brahmin community continue to perform the ritual of Samati Sadang which celebrates the coming of menarche. The wish that the young girl may lead a fertile life is incorporated in this ritual. Samati Sadang is conducted by a married male relative who has had a happy (fertile) life. The girl sits on banana leaves, eats raw egg prepared in ginger oil, and is given a milk bath. When the ritual is concluded, the entire family joins her in a feast celebrating menarche and her emergence as a mature female.

If such ceremonies existed in our culture, we would be campaigning to have them stopped. We would object to the practice and purpose of scarification, rubbing the genitals with nettles, and the emphasis on fertility. Our objections would be justified, since these ceremonies perpetuate the taboo on menstruating woman and narrowly define the role she is expected to play until the time when she comes to menopause. The absence of ritual, however, does not prove that the taboo is nonexistent.

In our culture, a young woman is left alone to do the best she can. Often she must find out about every aspect of menstruation for herself, from the ways in which menstrual flow is collected to the ways in which the experience of cyclicity is incorporated into a sense of self. And most crucial of all, since she is living in an environment which gives no outward sign that a menstrual taboo exists, she must learn about all its implications and the ways she must act to prevent its transgression.

Adults say, "Congratulations, today you are a woman." This is the ceremony practiced by members of our tribes. Adults applaud the appearance of fertility (which they mistakenly believe is simultaneous

with menarche) but fear its results. We herald the arrival of woman-
liness but fear women.

In some families a vestige of more elaborate ritual remains. Among
Jewish families, for example, it is customary to slap a young

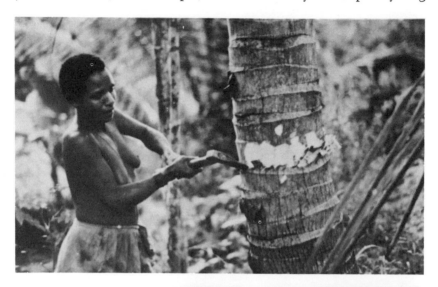

These two photographs
illustrate an unusual celebration of female puberty.
Among the Ilahita Arapesh
in New Guinea, the coconut
palm is symbolic of "things
male," while the coconut
itself symbolizes the female.

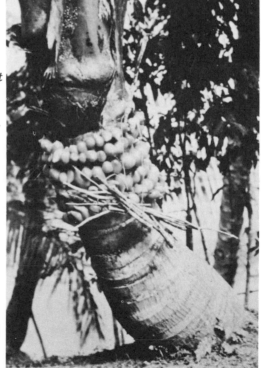

Above, a woman cuts a
superficial ring around the
tree, skin deep. Afterward,
the tree is decorated, as
seen in the photograph to
the right; strings of beautiful, inedible fruits are tied
around the wound and a
small bundle of kindling
wood is hung from them.
This ceremony is performed
to ensure that the tree will
produce bountifully.

woman's face on the day that menstruation begins. The women I have met who had this experience say they hadn't the vaguest notion of why their mothers slapped them. Many believed that it was a unique experience and the product of an aberration or a disturbed mother. Only one woman reported a different experience. She had a sense of tradition and positive feelings about her first menstruation. Her mother had taken her into the living room, and said, "As my mother did to me, as her mother did to her, so I do to you today." The mother then slapped her daughter across the face. When this woman grew up she said she felt proud to be menstruating and enjoyed a feeling of connection with her female ancestors—it gave her a sense of generational continuity which she, in turn, passed on to her daughter.

Pleasurable experiences of menarche are not common enough. For every woman responding to the menstrual survey who said menarche was a positive experience, another said it was negative; for every woman who said it was exciting, there was another who said it was

Navaho celebration of menarche

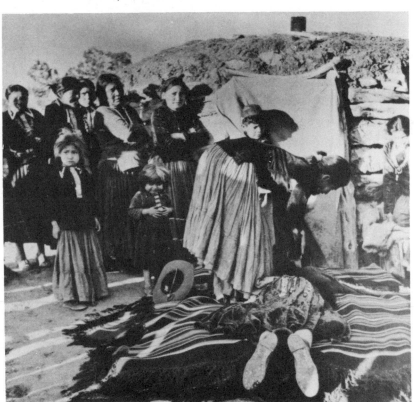

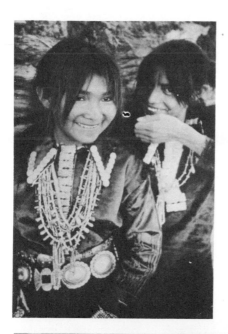
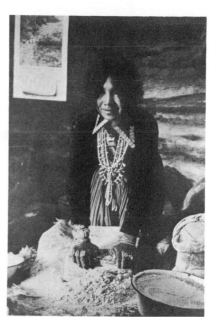
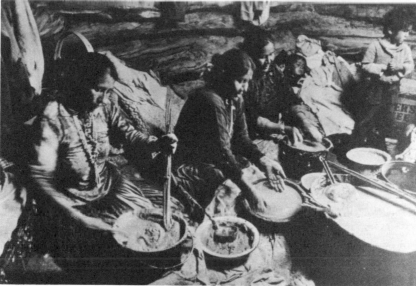
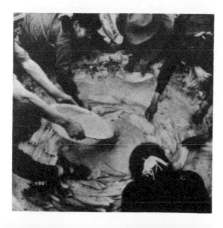
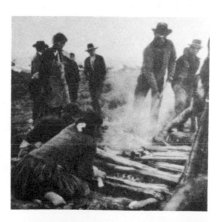

frightening. Twenty-three percent of the women remembered menarche as neutral; 59 percent said they had been adequately prepared, and 39 percent that preparation was inadequate. But only a quarter of the women understood the relationship between sex and reproduction when they began menstruating. Mothers and other educators all too often take a giant emotional leap backward at the sign of menarche. "It" is untouchable, and, in some sense, so is the young woman.

Adult avoidance of menarche takes many forms. Menstruation may be treated as a "simple" biological event. Presented as a more or less natural event, the hope is to defuse it of its complex meanings and to deny that it initiates a taboo which will be with the woman for the next thirty or forty years. This attempt at "naturalness" rarely succeeds. One handbook says: "A mother might want to reassure her daughter that despite its being somewhat of a nuisance, menstruation is an entirely healthy process and one that really makes it possible for her to function biologically as a woman."*[3] It strains the imagination to believe that a young woman would consider this kind of a message reassuring. Menstruation is labeled a nuisance, evidently the most positive description possible. Indeed, within the framework of the menstrual taboo, the monthly cycle is aptly described as a necessary evil—necessary so that women may bear children; evil for reasons left undisclosed or discussed.

This menstrual lesson is being repeated in hundreds of thousands of households, perhaps the very same dwellings in which the young woman learned in her childhood that having babies (preceded by that damned menstrual flow) would be her equivalent to her brother's penis.

> When a little girl asks her parents why her brother has a penis and she has none, she is usually told that when she is grown she will have both breasts and babies and the boy will not. This is usually sufficient reassurance of the equality of physical equipment simply because the real time lag involved is beyond the comprehension of small children.[4]

This excerpt from Judith Bardwick reads like a tale from a primer on penis envy. Bardwick, however, doesn't believe that little girls suffer from penis envy because, she says, little girls aren't terribly sexual and therefore don't mind that their brothers have a sexual organ and that they will "have" to wait until they grow up for a penis equivalent!

---

* Once again we see that biological "function" is restricted to maternity in the same way that social function is often restricted to maternity. The sexual implications of physical maturity as well as the emotional implications of cyclicity are absolutely ignored.

An ability to be satisfied with the promise of future gratification is difficult for adults; it is beyond the scope of children. A young girl is not reassured by such a statement but she may be effectively stopped from asking further questions. A child will doubtless continue to enjoy the pleasure of her clitoris while believing that adults consider this a secret pleasure and one that "doesn't count" in the way that having a penis or babies counts. She will understand that in the world of adults, producing children is somehow a sexual act and source of permissible sexual fulfillment, and she will years later learn that menarche is the sign that "adult" sexuality is now available to her.

The day finally comes when the young woman begins to menstruate. It is popularly believed that on this day she becomes fertile and sexual parity is achieved. Menarche therefore has been set up as a momentous event.

> During prepuberty menstruation is for many girls one of the important subjects of "secrets." The little friends observe the older girls with curiosity and envy, they respect, admire and pity them, and wonder in a strong spirit of competition whose turn will come next. This conscious and whipped-up expectation typically ends in great disappointment. The young girl hopes that with the onset of menstruation her role with regard to her environment will change and that she herself will experience something new and momentous. Above all, she hopes to be recognized as a grown-up and to acquire new rights. . . . Young girls who have reacted to the first menstruation with depressions often openly admit that they were previously informed about the facts and yet experienced a painful feeling of being surprised. . . . "Here is the longed-for, tremendous event, yet nothing has changed around me or inside me."*5

Young women may be disappointed at menarche because they have been given lessons which are from beginning to end filled with deception. The lies given to girl children and young women are outgrowths of a societal need to create a vulnerable creature who will have a weakened sense of her sexual identity and who will be forced to focus her striving for identity on men and on motherhood. She is taught to believe that she is sexually inadequate in comparison to men, but that men can save her and that motherhood will redeem her.

The biological event which heralds her potential motherhood is *not* a joyous event, however. Adults consider it unpleasant, messy, and downright unclean. This assessment of menstruation is yet another

---

* The tacit belief that menarche is a sexual event is understood in this extract from Deutsch. The classic responses to menarche and to "losing" one's virginity are so similar that they are virtually identical.

nail in the coffin of female self-respect. The one salvation, the one source of equality her body provides is bound up with something corrupt and tainted. This is the lesson of menarche, and disappointment is the mildest of responses.

> In all civilizations and still in our day, woman inspired man with horror; it is the horror of his own carnal contingence which he projects upon her. The little girl not yet in puberty carries no menace, she is under no taboo and has no sacred character. . . . But on the day she can reproduce, woman becomes impure. . . .[6]

Young women, of course, are not told, in so many words, that menarche is the entry into a life of impurity and corruption. In a culture where girls are sheltered from knowledge of their sexual organs and deprived of sexual equality, it is natural that they are also spared an analysis of the origins of sexual suppression and the genesis of the menstrual taboo. Young women are abandoned at menarche and their vulnerability is increased. Through this technique they are prepared for acceptance of the taboo and quickly learn of its nature. Deutsch feels that: "Menstruation is very often the one thing that the mother conceals from her children with particular discretion; it is a secret, and the idea of revealing it meets with great psychological resistance on her part. Many mothers find it much easier to talk with their daughters about conception, pregnancy, and birth than about menstruation."[7]

Some mothers are so uncomfortable with the subject of menstruation that they avoid telling their daughters anything at all. Others take refuge in overly scientific explanations of reproduction, as though science will come to the rescue, defuse the meaning of menstrual flow, and obscure the meaning of menstrual cyclicity. Occasionally, mothers are filled with horror toward their daughter's menstruation and communicate this quite directly.

I repeatedly asked my mother. . . . She repeatedly said, "Ask your cousin." (Cousin also gave me the inside info on Santa Claus and the Easter Bunny.) (v.p.r.)

It would have helped if my mother hadn't treated the subject so squeamishly by telling me only the causes and scientific facts that were far removed from my reality. "The shedding of the lining of the uterus" is a far cry from the reality that I was bleeding. . . . She couldn't understand why I was shocked or didn't connect that funny looking picture [of the reproductive organs] to the blood in my panties. (j.d.)

I wasn't even sure it was my period when I began to menstruate because it was brown and small in amount. I was scared to tell anyone. I thought something was wrong with me, until I asked my girl friend about it. She said not to worry about it because that's how her first period was, too. She said that the night before she got her first period she had eaten a caramel and she thought it came out the wrong opening. (D.J.H.)

I thought my first cycle was the only one I'd have. Imagine my shock to find this happens every month. (J.M.P.)

My mother almost overprepared me—I knew all the details about reproduction by about the fourth grade. But she always implied it was "no big deal," so when I started menstruating, I suppressed the excitement I felt. Unfortunately, this has caused problems! I never knew the woman was supposed to enjoy sex, and I had never heard of an orgasm 'til shortly after my first sexual experience. I think I knew the facts well enough, but sex was presented as reproduction rather than an emotional experience. My period seemed rather like cutting my toenails—just something that happens. I was excited, felt grown-up and "special," but I was ashamed of these feelings and can only vaguely remember them. (M.W.)

I expected to turn into a beautiful fairy princess—felt ugly when I did not. (B.P.)

I had no information whatsoever, no hint that anything was going to happen to me, and then to make everything nicer, I had been suffering from a severe kidney infection. When this mysterious gush of blood appeared, of course, I thought I was on the point of death from internal hemorrhage. . . .

What did my highly-educated mother do? She read me a furious lecture about what a bad, evil, immoral thing I was to start menstruating at the age of eleven! So young and so vile! Even after thirty years, I can feel the shock of hearing her condemn me for "doing" something I had no idea occurred. (H.M.L.)

Given this sort of response to menarche, it is hardly surprising that no special attention is paid to early or late menstruation; but for the individual girl, variations from the norm (twelve to thirteen years) can present serious problems. The normal range for onset of menstruation stretches from the ninth to the seventeenth year. Menarche at *any* age within this range is normal and perfectly healthy. For girls who begin to menstruate at the early end of this continuum and for those at the late end (and sometimes for their mothers as well), the experience may be filled with anxiety and feelings of vulnerability. Menarche is the "symbol" of womanhood—it is the focus of everyone's fears and fantasies about femininity, the young girl's as well as those of the adults around her.

I was tremendously relieved because I was the last of my group to start and had begun to wonder what was wrong with me. [Menarche at age fourteen.] (C.L.)

I began to feel left out because my friends had started and I hadn't. [Menarche at age thirteen.] (K.E.D.)

Absurdly enough, my starting later than most of my friends did affect me. I had trouble relating to boys until after I began to menstruate. I guess I felt "inadequate" if that's possible. [Menarche at age fourteen.] (L.E.)

The girl who comes to menarche late is relieved to find out that she too is a woman. Each year that passes after she reaches the average starting time is a year filled with worry that she will never "arrive." She may be relieved that she does not yet have to conform to the behavior appropriate for a "young lady," but she also feels left out and at a disadvantage with her friends of both sexes.

The girl who begins menstruation before the average age has another set of difficulties. She may enjoy the sense of superiority in "getting there first," but she will also feel the isolation of being there alone:

I was very sensitive about my early development as compared with my friends. I was ashamed of my body—felt like a cow. [Menarche at age ten.] (M.L.)

Adults often pay little attention to the variation in age at menarche and the particular blessings and problems for the individual young woman; however, her friends don't overlook these variations. The girl who has a late start may be pitied by her friends, yet they may also enjoy the advantages of knowing something she has yet to find out. The girl who begins before all her friends can be the object of resentment and jealousy.

The strength of such feelings is suggested in a short story by Grace Paley entitled "Faith in the Afternoon." The central character, Faith, is a grown woman living with her own family. She has just learned that a girlhood friend, Anita, is now getting a divorce:

Faith bowed her head in sorrow for Anita Franklin, whose blood when she was nine and three quarters burst from her to strike life and hope into the busy heads of all the girls in the fifth and sixth grades. Anita Franklin, she said to herself, do you think you'll make it all alone? How do you sleep at night, Anita Franklin, the sexiest girl in New Utrecht High?[8]

Faith's memory of her jealousy has endured for twenty years; Anita's divorce, some twenty years later, is seen as the fair comeuppance for having dared to be the sexiest kid in the class. Whatever the rewards of starting early, the penalties are at least as great.

The envy of friends toward the girl who comes to menarche earliest, their condescension toward the girl who is the last to menstruate, continue to affect the relationships of these people long after the event. The feelings and ideas of the girl who experiences a precocious or delayed menarche affect a young woman's idea of herself, her estimation of her femininity and sexiness, as well as her evaluation of her worth in relation to her friends—both girls and boys.

The girl who begins menstruating early may feel that she has received a special blessing (along with some special burdens) and the girl who is late may feel that she has been punished for a transgression (known only to herself). She and her friends will have no more clear idea of why menstruation begins and what accounts for the age of its initiation than do the adults who guide them. Cosmic forces are called upon to "explain" these events—events which are, in fact, absolutely earthly.

Avoidance of menstruation, inattention to menarche, leaves young women in a state of ignorance. Then fate is called in to explain the "unknowable." The timing of menarche is relegated to mystic powers, while the onset of fertility is said to be fixed at the onset of menstruation. Just as it is absurd to suggest the timing of menarche is a mystical event, it is false to say that fertility is present at menarche. The belief that menarche heralds the beginning of fertility is perpetuated because very few people pay attention to what is known of menstruation. M. F. Ashley Montagu has documented the period of adolescent sterility* which exists in all the cultures he studied.[9] For a year or two after menarche, most cycles occur *without* ovulation. In cultures where intercourse occurs in this postmenarchic interval, con-

---

* Most cycles are nonovulatory in the two years after menarche, but there is no way of predicting which cycles *will* include extrusion of an egg cell. Young women who are having intercourse would be risking pregnancy were they to avoid contraception during this interval.

ception rarely follows until a year or two years after menarche. Adolescent sterility is no more mystical in origin than the timing for menarche.*

Menstrual pain most often occurs in ovulatory cycles (see chapter 2). Most women, therefore, do not begin to experience cramping with menstruation until a year or more *after* menarche. The cause of dysmenorrhea is not known, but it is related to sex hormone levels (see chapter 2). Its existence is, unfortunately, well documented—as is the refusal of many adults to take it seriously:

What angers me most about my experience is my mother's (and others') attitude that dysmenorrhea is a natural, harmless occurrence and part and parcel of a woman's lot. From the onset of my period I suffered such pain, nausea and lightheadedness that I regularly missed a day or two of school. Many times I fainted on the way to the school nurse's office, twice almost falling down a flight of stairs. . . . Through all this my mother only allowed me to consult two doctors. . . . Both prescribed the same pill. Its only effect was to make me throw up sooner. . . . Most of my friends suffered almost as much as I did and received almost as little comfort. (M.L.F.)

Adults hide menstruation and hide from it. In most cases, this adult aversion increases a young woman's problems. Occasionally, she will capitalize on the embarrassment menstruation causes adults and use it to her advantage; most often, however, the pain overshadows the benefits.† She may sense the shame of adults about menstruation and make use of it, but she is less likely to grasp the severity of the menstrual taboo and the effects it has on her life. How can she, after all, appreciate the price she will pay as a result of being abandoned by her culture?

Deutsch suggested that disappointment and depression follow menarche because the world does *not* change for the young woman. The internal world most definitely does change with menarche, but the external world is made up of adults who steadfastly ignore what is happening. A basic change *has* taken place, yet the people closest to

---

* The discussion of Dr. Rose E. Frisch's work on critical weight is in chapter 2. There is one critical weight needed for the onset of menarche and a second for the onset of regular periods of ovulatory cycles.

† In a recent talk with several high-school girls, I learned that menstruation is still being used as a "manipulation." Knowing that their teachers suffer from menstrual "shyness," these young women look the teacher square in the eye and explain that work wasn't done or classes were missed because ". . . you know . . . I was menstruating." It works, they said, like a charm—especially if the teacher's a man.

the young woman pretend it is a minor event. Adults have prepared the girl for an event which does not take place: she does not "become" a woman at the first flow of menstrual blood. They have not prepared her for the changes of menstrual cyclicity which they do not want to believe exist. One result of this pretense and deception is the difficulty young women have in perceiving the cyclic nature of biological and emotional experience. Cyclicity is lost in the shuffle.

Menarche *is* a momentous event—but not because it is the day when a "girl becomes a woman" or because she is finally possessed of a penis equivalent. It is important because it is the culmination of the first cyclic rhythm of the sex hormone cycle. These cycles will include ovulation in the future and so contain the potential for fertility; but they are also at once—as they will continue to be for thirty or forty years—rhythmic changes which will underlie and shape her biological and emotional experience. One might guess that cyclic changes are ignored because they are considered trivial; yet they are by no means trivial.

When sex education courses are provided for young people, they generally include a film on the reproductive system in which the explanation of the menstrual cycle becomes the animated story of the sperm and the egg. This concentration on the physiology of menstruation often bores the audience, who know that their attention is being diverted from the more pressing issues of sexual life. The audience is perhaps less aware that by focusing on ovarian mechanisms the instructors are implying that this is the complete story of menstruation and that cyclic changes in emotion and attitude do not exist.

Education about menstruation presents a problem for parents; their usual response to menarche is shame, embarrassment, or anger. Adults know too well that being a woman includes qualities other than those needed to be a "good" wife and mother, as they also know that being sexual includes many levels of feeling—some of which are not "nice." They know that the goddess/princess fantasy has its opposite side. Menstruation is the reminder that being a woman "means" being a sinner—the bearer of a curse. Menstruation kindles the terror once felt by men at the sight of genital blood (a feeling they no longer consciously identify), and it reminds adults of both sexes of the grand and frightening powers of sexuality—powers which man has projected onto woman as her exclusive property. These are the powers signified by the first drop of menstrual blood.

Once upon a time there was a good little girl made of sugar and spice and everything nice. This little girl disappears at menarche and in her place stands a potentially fatal woman. All the curls, bows, and shiny patent-leather shoes once so adorable and innocent are seen in retrospect as forerunners of the charms and manipulations of the adult woman, who will seize the right man and "captivate" him.

In our society the young lady at menarche will spend years perfecting her ability to attract the male of the species. She will learn to develop her sexuality to secure a domestic life. Her sexuality is permissible only if it is used to attract a mate, to enable their union to bring forth young, and to keep the home fires burning while the children are being raised.

Female sexuality, of which menarche is the pre-eminent symbol, is suppressed and its existence denied except within the permitted channels of femininity. Sexual passion is not an attribute of femininity, nor is sexual expression (unless it is tied to domesticity and motherhood).*

Young women learn about the dark side of being female through a long, slow process. They learn that although menstruation is termed a simple, natural event it has a hidden meaning and is a source for feeling shame. What do young men feel when they learn about the existence of menstruation?

A number of males, friends and mates of the women who responded to the menstrual survey, gave their answers to the question: "Did your attitude toward girls change when you knew about menstruation?" Some were condescending:

I was glad I didn't have to put up with that and felt sorry for women because they did. (D.P.)

At first I was concerned, then very cautious, I was rather paternalistic. (J.H.)

Others were alienated or repelled:

It seemed strange—I didn't understand the physical reasons. I heard it was dirty. (D.W.D.)

It merely confirmed my attitude that girls were different and "mysterious." (C.J.A.)

* During this period of transition, women are no longer uniformly expected to use their sexuality in order to secure a nest for children. However, the conception of the nurturing woman and her opposite, the libertine, are still the predominant images of feminine sexuality. The former type is considered "safe" to men, the latter dangerous; the former hides menstruation, obeying the laws of taboo, while the latter is, of course, described as scarlet.

I thought it was messy and repulsive. (R.G.)

To the extent that a young man enjoys the powers assumed by his sex, he is likely to perceive the "symbol" of femininity as a touching or repellent weakness. De Beauvoir says: "Puberty takes on a radically different significance in the two sexes because it does not portend the same future to them. . . . Just as the penis derives its privileged evaluation from the social context, so it is the social context that makes menstruation a curse. . . . Femininity signifies alterity and inferiority. . . ."[10]

If a young man were not protected by the armor of sexual advantage he would have a different attitude toward menarche. In "The Resemblance Between a Violin Case and a Coffin," Tennessee Williams writes beautifully on this subject:

With her advantage of more than two years and the earlier maturity of girls, my sister moved before me into that country of mysterious differences where children grow up. And although we naturally continued to live in the same house, she seemed to have gone on a journey while she remained in sight. The difference came about more abruptly than you would think possible, and it was vast, it was like the two sides of the Sunflower River that ran through the town where we lived. On one side was a wilderness where giant cypresses seemed to engage in mute rites of reverence at the edge of the river, and the blurred pallor of the Dobyne place that used to be a plantation, now vacant and seemingly ravaged by some impalpable violence fiercer than flames, and back of this dusky curtain, the immense cotton fields that absorbed the whole visible distance in one sweeping gesture. But on the other side, avenues, commerce, pavements and homes of people: those two, separated by only a yellowish, languorous stream that you could throw a rock over. The rumbling wooden bridge that divided, or joined, those banks was hardly shorter than the interval in which my sister moved away from me. Her look was startled, mine was bewildered and hurt. Either there was no explanation or none was permitted between the one departing and the one left behind. The earliest beginning of it that I can remember was one day when my sister got up later than usual with an odd look, not as if she had been crying, although perhaps she had, but as though she had received some painful or frightening surprise, and I observed an equally odd difference in the manner toward her of my mother and grandmother. She was escorted to the kitchen table for breakfast, as though she were in danger of toppling over on either side, and everything was handed to her as though she could not reach for it. She was addressed in hushed and solicitous voices, almost the way that docile servants speak to an employer. I was baffled and a little disgusted. I received no attention at all, and the one or two glances given me by my sister had a peculiar look of resentment in them. It was as if I had struck her in the night before and given her a bloody nose or a black eye, except that she wore no bruise, no visible injury, and there had been no altercation between us in recent days. I spoke to her several times, but for some reason she ignored my remarks, and when I became irritated and yelled at her, my grandmother suddenly reached over and twisted my ear, which was one of the few times that I can remember when she ever offered me more than the gentlest reproach. It was a Saturday morning, I remember, of a hot yellow day and it was the hour when my sister and I would ordinarily take to the streets on our wheels. But the custom was now disregarded. After breakfast my sister appeared somewhat strengthened but still alarmingly pale and silent as ever. She was then escorted to the parlor and encouraged to sit down at the piano. She spoke in low whimpering tones to my grandmother who adjusted the piano stool very carefully and placed a cushion on it and even turned the pages of sheetmusic for her as if she were incapable of finding the place for herself. She was working on a simple piece called *The Aeolian Harp*, and my grandmother sat beside her while she played, counting out the tempo in a barely audible voice, now and then reaching out to touch the wrists of my sister in order to remind her to keep them arched. Upstairs my mother began to sing to herself which was something she only did when my father had just left on a long trip with his samples and would not be likely to return for quite a while, and my grandfather, up since daybreak, was mumbling a sermon to himself in the study. All was peaceful except my sister's face. I did not know whether to go outside or stay in. I hung around the parlor a little while, and finally I said to Grandmother, Why can't she practice later? As if I had made some really brutal remark, my sister jumped up in tears and fled to her upstairs bedroom. What was the matter with her? My grandmother said, Your sister is not well today. She said it gently and gravely, and then she started to follow my sister upstairs, and I was deserted. I was left alone in the very uninteresting parlor. The idea of riding alone on my wheel did not please me for often when I did that, I was set upon by the rougher boys of the town who called me Preacher and took a particular delight in asking me obscene questions that would embarrass me to the point of nausea. . . . In this way was instituted the time of estrangement that I could not understand.[11]

With the coming of menarche young women learn too little about what is actually occurring within their bodies, the changes that are occurring in their pattern of feeling, and the changing attitudes of those who view them. They do learn that the privilege of acting the way they feel—climbing trees, playing baseball, hanging out with boys—is taken away at menarche. This is the time to grow up, the time to shape us as a feminine creature. For many, menarche is accompanied with a realistic feeling of lost freedom and pleasure which adds to the sense of abandonment shared by all young women at this time.

Menarche—Its Relationship to Behavior

A veil comes down between the young woman and her mates who are male. On her side, the veil covers a diminished figure, but on the far side of the veil are privileged beings who enjoy far greater freedom and opportunity—or so we believe. Thirty-two percent of the women responding to the menstrual survey, for example, reported that after menarche they felt that their status had been diminished. The majority of these women felt a loss of self-esteem and at the same time believed that the power of their male classmates had increased. This situation is surely reinforced by all the young men who now, suddenly, feel either repelled or sorry for the young women. While the abrupt change in status contributes to the malaise of adolescence for women, this changing status makes the stresses of adolescence much more bearable for most men.

Mercifully, adolescence passes and with it the intense confusion and disruption of sudden dramatic changes. The conflicts experienced during puberty and adolescence, of course, linger even though their intensity lessens, and the ways in which conflicts are resolved shape the character of adults. The paradoxical role of the female—the hormonal changes of menarche and menstruation, the pain and the blood—is accepted (in some fashion) whether or not an individual consciously thinks about any of these issues.

> But what is menstruation on the physiological and psychological levels? It is the beginning of emphatic periodicity in the girl's life—the starting of regular hormonal changes that we know are influential in mood states, in emotionality and its management, in general body tone, in water retention by body tissue, and in other physiologic and psychic conditions. The menarche introduces the peculiar female condition in which the whole body system is subject to regular periodic transformation—a condition unlike any of the equally significant changes a boy experiences at puberty.
>
> . . . This regular fluctuation in the bodily system—unique in the phenomena of normal physiology—adds special conflicts to the already

problem-ridden process of developing a stable self-concept at adolescence. It will, I think, alter both the process and the final outcome of the adolescent search for self.[12]

A young woman experiences sudden highs and lows, she may burst into tears for "no good reason." She becomes a stranger to herself, while to adults she is simply "passing through a stage." No one teaches the young woman about the changes that are taking place— no one wants to know about them.

This young woman coming to adolescence has no tools to use for gaining insight and self-understanding. She begins to believe these changes are happening *to* her, that the identity she possessed prior to menarche is being stripped away, and that she has no control over its loss and nothing with which to replace it. She becomes a mystery to herself as unknown forces present in almost every experience take possession of her body and spirit.

Menstrual cycle changes, for example, may affect the young woman's performance in school. Katharina Dalton studied the effects of the paramenstrum (described as the last few days preceding and the first few days of menstrual flow) on school behavior.[13] In one study she found that almost 20 percent of high-school girls do more poorly on examinations taken in the premenstrual week (including the first two days of flow). During this interval, exam scores are reduced by about five points compared with results of tests taken at other times of the cycle. If the examination is of minor importance to the overall grade, the score is inconsequential and may even go unnoticed. However, if a major examination like the SAT's is taken during the paramenstrum, this loss in score can have a profound effect on a young woman's future.

Dalton also studied records of punishments students incurred by breaking boarding-school rules. She correlated these records with dates of menstrual onset kept by the boarding-school health service and found that in more than half the cases, punishment occurred following infractions committed by girls who were in their paramenstrum.

Dalton attributes each of these effects to an underlying slowdown in reaction time during the paramenstrual interval. This leads to a blurring of thought processes in the first case and to an inefficiency when covering up misdeeds in the second. It is not that young women engage in misconduct more frequently before menstruation, she suggests, but that they are slower to cover their tracks and therefore more likely to be found out.

In either case, a young woman is not likely to understand that her behavior is being influenced by hormonal and other bodily changes related to menstruation. She may feel victimized by bad luck or some other version of loss of control over her environment. These experiences will only add to all the others (including the overriding lack of attention paid to menstruation and all its ramifications) which make her feel insecure and unable to rely upon herself.

The young woman who suffers from menstrual pain will, of course, have more than a clue about the relationship between menstruation and poor test scores, but she may nevertheless feel victimized. Menstrual problems are not generally considered legitimate by physicians, teachers, adults at large, and in many cases by young women themselves.*

In exceptional cases, adults do understand some of the effects of menstruation. But it is rare to meet an adult who gives a younger person a sense of knowing the full range of menstrual experience or even acknowledges the existence of a menstrual cycle. A young woman finds it hard to learn about cyclicity from the messages of her own body in a world where menstruation is taboo, where cyclicity and flow are buried and the desire to make these events nonexistent is strong. She grows to mistrust her body. If she listens to its messages, they seem erratic, confused, and mysterious. If she develops a sensitivity to cyclicity, she is left alone with it and may come to feel that she is imagining things rather than correctly perceiving what is really happening. Douvan says: "Since internal cues vary widely and appear unstable, the girl will come to rely more heavily than the normal boy on external cues and the expectations of significant others—on feedback from an audience—as anchors for her self-definition."[14]

The forces that converge upon a young woman at this time of her life do not exist in a vacuum. They are part of an environment in which the definition of femininity and the correct attitudes toward menstruating women are clearly defined.

> Many women will, of course, say that the chief end of women is not necessarily to marry and breed children. While at the present time the number of women so exceeds that of men that there are many of the former who are forced to this conclusion, the fact remains that the great majority of women must make their chief aspiration the cares of

* I remember only one case in which a professor made room at the top of a final examination for a statement of how his students were feeling that day. As it happened I was feeling fine and did not learn how he interpreted the other responses; but my feeling was that, unlike many other teachers, he would take the answers seriously into account when scoring the exam.

wifehood and motherhood. Let those who are sure that this lot will never be theirs undertake anything they desire. If they want to attain to high effort they may hurt themselves, but the nation will not greatly suffer, neither will the well-being of future generations be affected. Throw open to them all doors that they may achieve greatness, and do noble service for mankind, even though they destroy themselves by their efforts. Let us honor them for the sacrifice they make even though, at first, malignant fate forced this destiny upon them.

Only we must insist as we have the good of the nation at heart, that no woman shall enter upon these absorbing intellectual pursuits in the critical, formative period between advent and full establishment of womanhood.[15]

Thus, in 1892, Webster insisted that a young woman not try to define herself during the years between puberty and maturity—she would find her identity as she took on the roles of wife and mother. Such an admonishment might be perceived as an intriguing bit of cultural history, of biting importance in our grandmothers' time but not for us, and surely not for the young approaching menarche today. But 1973 brought the following message:

In general, the whole range of society, marriage and careers—and thus the social order—will be best served if most men have a position of economic superiority over the relevant women in the community, and if in most jobs the sexes tend to be segregated by either level or function.

These practices are seen as oppressive by some; but they make possible a society in which men can love and respect women and treat them humanely.[16]

Young women formed in the image given them by men will be less likely to perceive the feminine role as oppressive than women given an alternative, a means of defining their view of femininity themselves. With time, however, experience leads women to review the manner and matter of woman's education. The lessons these men propound are only reflections of widely held beliefs that are still very much alive. Webster, for example, "permits" women to engage in nondomestic, serious pursuits if they cannot do better. Today this message is heard again at menopause, when reproductive function ceases and women can no longer "do better"—only then is it safe for women to pursue nondomestic aims. Gilder embroiders this theme by assuring women that love, respect, and even humane treatment are theirs in exchange for human oppression. The threat is clear: if a woman refuses to accept a lowly status during her fertile years, she will lose love, and while she may gain self-respect she will lose the respect of men. This is a choice that a man is never asked to make, so he cannot appreciate the price it involves for a woman. As M. F. Ashley Montagu points out: "Men have been jealous of woman's ability to give birth to children and they have been jealous of their ability to menstruate; but men have not been content with turning these capacities into disabilities, for they have surrounded the one with handicapping rituals and the other with taboos which, in most cases amount to punishments."[17]

At menarche, a young woman learns that she is a tabooed creature. She has grasped the rules of the game, through her mother and teachers, who very often will avoid talking about menstruation or the menstrual cycle and thereby have denied her the help she needs for incorporating this new experience into her life and conception of herself. Each of us in our silence about menstruation encourages the young woman to believe the taboo is just. She will be subject to this taboo and to the feelings of inferiority it engenders until she comes to menopause. By the time the curse is lifted, her belief in herself will be almost too fragile to be reclaimed. The psychoanalyst Clara Thompson observed that:

> She was taught to be ashamed of menstruation. It was something to be concealed and any accident leading to its discovery was especially humiliating. In short, womanhood began with much unpleasantness. It was characterized by feelings of body shame, loss of freedom, loss of equality with boys, and loss of the right to be aggressive. The training in insincerity especially about her sexual being and sexual interest has undoubtedly contributed much to woman's diminished sense of self. When something so vitally a part of her must be denied, it is not a great step further to deny the whole self.[18]

At menopause a woman is expected to become more independent, even though she may have lived for thirty or forty years following the instructions meted out at menarche: depend on others. If she has followed her early instruction zealously, she will have the most meager sense of self-definition upon which to call at menopause. When a female agrees to become a "good" woman, she pays the price of loss of self throughout her life.

8

Woman
in the Moon

Children look into the night sky and see the face of the man
in the moon; adults look at the television screen and see earth men
walking the moon's surface. Despite the colonization of the moon's
surface, it continues to shine its light as the symbol of woman, the
female, the other.

> The sun is the constant and reliable source of light and heat, but the
> moon is changeable. . . . The darkness falls at the setting of the sun.
> Surely the moon should then rise and give us light throughout the dark
> hours, but she is not to be relied on. . . . In these unaccountable
> qualities of the moon, man has seen a symbol of woman's nature which
> to him appears erratic, changeable . . . not to be relied on.[1]

Man has taken for himself the symbol of the sun, the sustainer of
life, while woman has been symbolized in the world of darkness and
unpredictability. The night world and the light that shines upon it are
filled with danger and mystery; these are the attributes man has seen
in his sister, mother, and mate.

Where men have found it useful, they have unlocked the secrets of
the moon: sailors and fishermen needing to know the laws of the
tides learned to chart them. More recently, men have fulfilled their
need to travel to the moon and completely master its mystery. But
the laws underlying the cycles of menstruation which man has
metaphorically bound to the moon have not been explained, nor has
explanation been sought, because man has kept the image of woman
filled with mystery. By the time she is adult, woman has thoroughly

learned the perceptions of men and has incorporated the view that she is mysterious and unknowable—even to herself. Men and women believe that woman is, by nature, an alien and has always been so.

For centuries men have observed and taught that woman is a creature beyond human understanding. To Freud, who dared to travel into psychic worlds previously uncharted, woman remained a mystery and the mother goddess was beyond understanding. As he charted unconscious terrain, woman was given the place of the shadow; she had no existence of her own. But history gives evidence that at one time the image of woman wielded power equal to that of the male gods who came after her.

> . . . Ishtar the moon goddess of Babylon was thought to be men-struating at the full moon, when the Sabbattum or evil day of Ishtar was observed. The word Sabbattum comes from Sa-bat and means Heart-rest; it is the day of rest which the moon takes when full, for at that time it is neither increasing nor decreasing. On this day, which is the forerunner of the Sabbath, it was considered unlucky to do any work or to eat cooked food or to go on a journey. These are the things that are prohibited to menstruating women. On the day of the moon's menstruation everyone, whether man or woman, was subject to similar restrictions, for the taboo of the menstruating woman was on all. The Sabbath was at first observed only once a month, later it was kept at each quarter of the moon's phases.[2]

The Babylonian Sabbattum was an evil day, but it was the day of "Heart-rest" as well. While the menstrual taboo was present in that culture, the spirit which symbolized menstruating woman was honored and the fears of men were brought under control. Woman and the moon were "knowable"—and both were respected.*

We know little about the everyday life of those cultures where women were honored and both men and women showed equal re-spect to the menstruating goddess. But surely this kind of equality reflects a culture with vastly different beliefs from our own. Certainly, it differs from our culture where the brunt of taboo is directed toward women, who must bear the largest part of the resulting psychic effects.

In cultures where menstruating women are not honored but feared,

---

* The Sabbath of the Judaic and Christian God is a day of work-rest honoring the spirit which created the world. This male figure did not give birth to the world—he built it. His labor is respected in the Sabbath and his vengeance averted by the homage paid on this day. Even though the evil of menstruation remains, the honor of the rest has disappeared.

women are unable to trust themselves and therefore also unable to trust one another.

> In Tibet each tent dwelling is built around a central hearth. This hearth is sacred as it is the dwelling place of the gods and spirits. . . . Because of it the women who do not belong to the family, or who are not intimate friends, may not enter a strange tent. In Tibet . . . a woman is regarded as an impure creature. . . . In her impure [menstruating] state she might anger the gods and spirits and thus evoke the family's ruin.
>
> In Tibet, as well as in China and among so many other peoples, the women are thought to bring bad luck. Since there is no way of knowing what condition a strange woman is in and whether she might not be hostile to the family, she is never permitted in the kitchen or tent.[3]

In the cultures of pre-revolutionary Tibet, women did not trust other women to enter their homes or their kitchens (unless they were close friends or were related). In contemporary Western culture, the gods and spirits certainly do not reside in the kitchen. In fact, the kitchen is so far removed from the sacred life that it is now the appropriate domain for women's social life. The world of the kitchen does not "count"—but in the worlds outside the hearth, women don't trust one another and think of each other as dangerous and unreliable. In the areas that our culture labels important and consequential, women are still outcasts, believed capable of undermining positive values. This can be seen quite clearly in the world of art—for our culture, the domain of the transcendent spirit. Woman's "inferiority" has kept her from achieving a vaunted role in Western art. Precedent for this assessment is found in at least one more primitive culture, as Margaret Mead has shown:

> All that is strange, that is uncharted and unnamed—unfamiliar sounds, unfamiliar shapes—these are forbidden to women, whose duty is to guard their reproductivity closely and tenderly. This prohibition cuts them off from all speculative thought and likewise from art, because among the Arapesh, art and the supernatural are part and parcel of each other. . . . The feeling against woman's participation in art and in the men's cult is one and the same; it is not safe, it would endanger the women themselves, it would endanger the order of the universe within which men and women and children live in safety.[4]

With the development of more sophisticated (though far from perfect) means of birth control, the idea that women must tenderly guard their reproductive potential has become outmoded. However, as long as woman menstruates she is "unsafe," and the universe must still be protected from her powers as she continues to need protection from herself.*

Through the development of modern-day myths, female art is said to reflect female truths, which are, by definition, minor and partial. Even in the arts that honor the anti-hero, only men are imbued with the power to make substantial statements. As Georg Simmel puts it:

> The requirements of art, patriotism, morality in general and social ideas in particular, correctness in practical judgment and objectivity in theoretical knowledge, the energy and profundity of life—all these categories which belong as it were in their form and their claims to humanity in general, but in the actual historical configuration they are masculine throughout. Supposing that we describe these things, viewed as absolute ideas, by the single word "Objective" we then find that in the history of our race the equation, objective = masculine, is a valid one.[5]

Art, which is subjective in its creation, is objective in its definition and evaluation. The moment subjectivity is given form, whether in art or ideas, its *product* is in the possession of the masculine world. The value of work done by women artists is questioned, while it is a matter of faith that women make formidable contributions to the creation of important works when they play the part of muse or helpmate.

Among the legions who were (and are) the typists, copyists, or ego massagers of "important" men are some who were enraged or burned out by the job, while other women have reveled in the flattery so often bestowed on the woman "behind" the power. In the latter cases, these women have incorporated men's estimate of female worth so thoroughly that they believe complete self-fulfillment comes through service to the artist/man.

This is the background from which any woman comes to the work of creation. The world of men has decreed that on her own she can produce nothing of great merit. A woman angered by this contemptuous attitude toward her sex might choose in creation to call solely upon that which is unique, cyclic, "other" in her nature—as though daring men to criticize the female principle in its most pure

* At menopause, when a woman is considered no longer dangerous and is free to join the men's cult in our society without reprisal, she must begin to acquire the knowledge and skills needed for full participation (see also chapter 9).

form. Or she might choose to bury what is unique to her sex and dare men to take her work seriously on "equal," that is, objective terms.

The work of the first woman, of course, will be dismissed (after appropriate bows to the "cause" of womanhood) because it is too "subjective." The work of the second will be appraised with relative coolness. Men will take this work seriously, but they will not find it of equal *value*. In this case they are making a correct judgment for the wrong reasons. Had they bothered to take the work of the first woman seriously they might, with equal justice, have found it suffering from a similar excess (though one of opposite direction). Like the work of a man who obsessively dwells on manliness or the work of a man who wishes to suppress his manhood, the work of these women will for identical reasons fail to achieve greatness. To deny the self uses energy, energy that is desperately needed to push oneself to the outer limits of courage and capability. It is this precious energy that women waste before setting out to dispel man's notions of art: ". . . it is fatal for anyone who writes to think of their sex. It is fatal to be a man or a woman pure and simple; one must be woman-manly or man-womanly."[6]

And so there is a third choice for the woman confronting the moment of creation. She may use all of herself, her cycles, her moods, and her linearity to one end. As Virginia Woolf went on to write in *A Room of One's Own:*

> Some collaboration has to take place in the mind between the woman and the man before the act of creation can be accomplished. Some marriage of opposites has to be consummated. The whole of the mind must lie wide open if we are to get the sense that the writer is communicating his experience with perfect fullness. There must be freedom and there must be peace. . . .[7]

It is freely acknowledged that any man who creates is making at least minimal use of that within him which is feminine. How perverse that femininity in expression is acceptable only when it passes through the body of a man; when a woman expresses herself in the fullness of that self, she is assailed for revealing her weakness and showing her fatal flaw to the world.

Menstruation and menopause are the sign and symbol of that which is decidedly unique in woman. These are the events which men call upon when they wish to "explain" the source of female subjectivity and codify the "fact" of female weakness. These, then, are the phenomena which men have used to "prove" that women cannot, *by nature,* make any creation of importance (except, of course, that of the next generation). We are told that the work of the ovaries is an inherent disability, but we are also told that it is more than compensation for anything that man can do. Neither men nor women are deceived by this tale. Cynthia Ozick has commented:

> Perhaps it is a compliment to a woman of no gifts to say of her in compensation, "Ah, well, but she has made a child." But that is a cheap and slippery mythology, and a misleading one. It induces the false value of self-inflation in mediocre women. It is scarcely our duty to compliment the mediocre for their mediocrity when we are hardly employed enough in celebrating the gifted for their gifts, wrung out by the toil of desire and imagination. It takes something away from Yeats to compare a mediocre child—and most children, like most parents, *are* mediocre—with *Sailing to Byzantium.* But it is just as irrelevant to compare a brilliant child with a brilliant poem. Biology is *there:* it does not need our praise, and if we choose to praise it, it is blasphemous to think we are praising not God but ourselves.[8]

Yet in the domain of woman, biology is not "there," it is hither and yon. We are, alternately, blessed madonnas and the cursed who bleed from the uterus only to "dry up" at menopause. As we career off each pole we are dunned by laws telling us the "proper" evaluation of each event.

In adolescence the laws of femininity are spelled out and the laws of the menstrual taboo instilled into the feelings of every young woman and man. The price paid by young women is high, and it keeps escalating with each new decade of life. The longer we live, the more opportunity we have to develop, the more we give up in exchange for conforming to the feminine role and the proscriptions of the taboo.*

The longer women live, however, the greater their opportunity to perceive that what one feels is different from what one has been told to feel or told did not even exist. As women encourage one another to speak out about what they have felt and seen, we will learn more about the experience of being female. Already women are beginning to see a new picture of feminine identity. This, on occasion, includes an entirely new evaluation of the menstrual cycle.

---

* The rewards given to women in exchange for obedience to taboo and sexual role, while of potentially great magnitude, are being steadily devalued both by individual women and the culture at large—bearing great numbers of children is no longer socially acceptable, and marriage is followed by divorce at an ever-increasing rate.

To the extent that it [menstruation] is regular and recurrent, I think it is a great psychological advantage to women. That there is something cyclical which will continue to happen to you when everything else can be blown to hell in the time of a month. I sometimes think men must envy this reassurance in women. (E.M.H.)

Monthly flow of blood and monthly cycles of feeling are experienced during each year of a woman's life between menarche and menopause (except during pregnancy). Recurrent bleeding is not likely to be a reassuring source of feminine identity because it has for so long been the symbol of woman's impurity, the sign of her shame. What of cyclicity? Is it also subject to a negative evaluation?

It is, I feel, a rather common, if crude joke among men that when they are confronted by a cranky or irritable woman they often shrug off her actions by saying, "She's on the rag," or she's "OTR."

Some guys even jokingly use this as an excuse for their own irritation. . . . In a fraternity I pledged at Purdue University, anyone in a bad mood who did not want to be disturbed would hang a sign on the door with the Greek letters O[omega] T[tau] R[rho]. . . . (D.N.F.)

Bitchiness as an aspect of the menstrual cycle would seem to be well documented and apparently quite "acceptable." D.N.F. recounts an anecdote that confirms this and also suggests the role of projection as a way of maintaining the taboo. Women are "naturally" bitchy. But when men feel this way, they find it comfortable to project it onto the female—perpetuating the illusion that "bitchiness," merely a transient experience, is alien to them, while to a woman it is second nature.

Other aspects of cyclicity are not as well documented, perhaps because they do not fit into the accepted notions of woman-the-terror. There is an absence of anecdote about other phases of the cycle as there is an absence of wide-ranging reports from women about the cycle. All eyes have been focused where the taboo suggests we look—at the time of flow.

The Menstrual Cycle—Its Relationship to Behavior

In recent years, social scientists have begun to study the menstrual cycle. In this country their research is generally done on college campuses among small groups of women (a fact that has led more than one scientist to say that research into the human psychology has given us the psychology of the college sophomore). The findings of these studies may best be considered preliminary and their importance rests on the fact that any investigations were carried out in an attempt to uncover some aspect of the female cyclic experience.

The psychologists Ivey and Bardwick wanted to study mood changes throughout the menstrual cycle to see whether or not a distinct emotional cycle exists which parallels the pattern of recurring hormonal change.[9] Twenty-six college students at two points in their menstrual cycles (once during the expected ovulatory period and once again just before menstrual flow) were asked to relate some past incident—*any* memory that spontaneously came to mind. The investigators studied the answers given during two complete cycles to see whether or not a particular pattern emerged. These are some of the responses they received:

> Talk about my trip to Europe. It was just the greatest summer of my life. We met all kinds of terrific people everywhere we went and just the most terrific things happened.

> Talk about my brother and his wife. I hated her. I just couldn't stand her mother. I used to do terrible things to separate them.

> We just went to Jamaica and it was fantastic. The island is so lush and green and the water is so blue. . . . The place is so fertile and the natives are just so friendly.

> I'll tell you about the death of my poor dog. . . . Oh, another memorable event, my grandparents died in a plane crash. It was my first contact with death and it was very traumatic for me. . . .

> We took out skis and parked them on top of the car and then we took off for up north. We used to go for long walks in the snow and it was really just great, really quiet and peaceful.

> . . . came around a curve and did a double flip and landed upside down. I remember the car coming down on my hand and slicing it right open and all this blood was all over the place. Later they thought it was broken because every time I touched my finger it felt like a nail was going through my hand.

In each pair of anecdotes, the first statement was given near the time of ovulation and the second near the anticipated time of flow. The pattern of responses is overwhelmingly evident—optimistic and life-affirming thoughts spontaneously arise near ovulation, while more morbid memories spring to consciousness near menstruation. In the midst of this study, the response pattern was so obvious and uniform that Bardwick was startled when one "ovulatory" woman began talking about an unhappy memory. A week later the woman returned and told Bardwick that menstrual flow had already begun—more than a week before it was expected. What had at first seemed like an unusual response at ovulation became, in retrospect, a prototype response at menstruation.

Further analysis of the answers showed that women felt the greatest sense of self-esteem near ovulation when they also felt most competitive. Aggressive feelings peaked in the period just before the onset of flow. When discussing the results of this study in *Psychology of Women*, Bardwick mentions that she was initially confused by the women who were most competitive near ovulation but most aggressive near menstruation. Weren't these two feelings just different aspects of an identical state? Eventually she realized that the contradiction was in her mind, not in the experience of the women she studied. She had been so steeped in the cultural assessment that a competitive woman is an aggressor that she had not seen what was right before her. Competition, she learned, and especially what one might label healthy competition, arises from the feeling that one can actually accomplish something; and this in turn stems from feelings of self-esteem rather than from aggressive needs.

The evidence in this investigation indicates a trend of astounding uniformity. Ovulation is associated with underlying optimism, the premenstrual period with underlying pessimism. The latter observation conforms to the accepted belief that menstruation is a negative experience. But this is just one aspect of the cycle, which contains *all* variations of feeling, each of equal importance in a woman's experience.* The days when a woman is predisposed to see the world colored with a rosy tint have as much bearing on her experience as the days when the edges of the world are blue. The cyclic alterations in feeling appear to be shared by most, if not all, women. "As psychologists we would expect to find strong individual differences in reaction during the menstrual cycle. Instead, in almost all of our subjects, we found the consistent and significant mood swings characteristic of a particular menstrual cycle phase. . . ."†[10]

* The assumption that every aspect of the cycle is equally important is based on a rather idealized vision. In fact, most aspects of the cycle are unnoticed, while great attention is paid only to the negative changes sometimes associated with the premenstrual interval.
† In this study individual variations are at a minimum. As Bardwick suggests, most psychological studies give evidence of wide-ranging variations of experience. Usually only the major trend is studied, and the variations are ignored.

Cyclic changes of mood paralleling the cyclic alterations in the levels of estrogen and progesterone may be a constant in the life of menstruating women. The magnitude of the cyclic peaks and valleys, of course, varies substantially. For some women these changes will be infinitesimal; for others they will be immense. But for most women the cyclic alterations in mood will fall somewhere in between these extremes.

A cyclic undercurrent to emotional perceptions is a unique experience affecting women only in the years of menstruation. It influences the way a woman perceives herself, the world she inhabits, and the people she knows. The *manner* in which cyclic variations influence behavior is much less clear, but it seems obvious that the greater the magnitude of variation in feeling, the more likely it is to influence behavior.

Almost every study of the behavioral aspects of the menstrual cycle has concentrated on the time of menstruation. This reflects the cultural bias of experimenters, since menstruation is generally considered the most important aspect of the cycle and the remaining variations relatively unimportant. In her book *The Menstrual Cycle*, Dalton concentrates on the ways in which behavioral change correlates with hormonal change during the few days before flow and the first few days of flow (she calls this time the paramenstrum). When combining her findings with the observations of her colleagues, she reports that, in the following categories, *more than half* the women studied were in a paramenstrum:

Newly convicted prisoners*
Disorderly prisoners*
Women asking for a physician's housecall
Accident admissions
Employees reporting sick*
Cases of acute mental distress
Hospital admissions for acute medical and surgical emergencies
Viral and bacterial infections
Mothers of sick children
Attempted or successful suicides* [11]

This should be kept in mind when reading about the findings of other studies reported in my book. As findings filter down into more widely read vehicles, the generalization level increases and the frequent exceptions are overlooked.
* When the *total* number of women in each of these categories is compared with the total number of men who would be placed in each category, *men* far outnumber women.

In many cases the studies from which these findings are drawn were carried on in almost anecdotal fashion, or the number of subjects asked was very small. For example, Dalton studied the menstrual history of 84 women who were admitted to London hospitals, 91 children whose mothers brought them for treatment of minor illness, 156 newly convicted prisoners, and 94 prisoners punished for creating disorder. The results of these studies should be approached with caution and might be best considered as an indication of trends which have yet to be confirmed.

These studies *suggest* that during the paramenstrum (when hormonal levels are at their low point), some negative alterations in behavior increase. In each category summarized in the list above, the number of women in their paramenstrum is *twice* as high as the number of women at any other time of the menstrual cycle. The trend indicates that the menstrual cycle phase does have a bearing on behavior, and women in the paramenstral portion of the cycle make up at least 50 percent of the total.*

While these studies cannot be considered definitive, the trends they uncover do provide us with some valuable information. For example, one item on Dalton's list, based on an investigation conducted by P. C. B. and I. L. MacKinnon, concerns bacterial and viral infections.[12] They did postmortems on forty-seven women. After analyzing the endometrial tissue, they were able to compare the time of death to the phase of menstrual cycle. Only two of the forty-seven women died during the follicular stage of their cycle; the rest had been in the luteal phase. (The majority of deaths had occurred while women were in the middle portion of the luteal phase.) These researchers concluded: "Planned operations, especially of the major variety . . . should be carried out in the follicular phase of the cycle."

In some hospitals (although none to my knowledge in the United States), the time of cycle often decides the scheduling of nonemergency surgery. A lowered resistance to infection might lead to the development of post-operative complications and present a greater risk to health than the surgical procedure or the initial cause for surgery. Not long ago I was scheduled for minor gynecological surgery. When the physician gave me a date for the procedure, I asked him (after consulting my menstrual calendar) to change it. He wanted to know

---

* Time of cycle is the only variable studied in any of these categories. If the actions of women were evenly distributed over the entire cycle, we would expect to find 25% of the total number of women in each phase of cycle. Instead, we find 50% (or more) grouped in the paramenstral phase and the remaining 50% scattered over the other three quarters of the cycle.

why. I explained that the day he suggested coincided with the para-menstrum, and I wished to change the date of surgery to a time outside this interval. While he agreed to change it, he did so with a slight tone of forced acceptance, rather as though I had said my astrologer hadn't found the day auspicious. Evidently the research done by his peers wasn't "important" enough to convince him that menstruation was something other than a minor annoyance.*

Many women have noticed that during the premenstrual week they feel as if they need unusual amounts of extra rest and sleep. If this aspect of the menstrual cycle is ignored along with the denial of the cycle's existence, infection becomes much more likely. The cautionary tales of the old wives—"Don't wash your hair, don't take a bath," and so on—have been tossed aside. While in detail these predictions were wrong (bathing doesn't cause colds and so forth), in spirit they were correct: it *is* wise to take extra precautions just prior to menstruation in order to avoid illness.

Dalton's observations about these findings take them out of the realm of mysterious and cosmic occurrence. The greater proportion of arrests for criminal conduct and punishments of criminal misbehavior during the paramenstrum can be traced to the same source suggested for increased misbehavior among schoolgirls discussed in the preced-ing chapter. The activities in question do *not* increase during the paramenstrum, she suggests, but only the clumsiness with which they are carried out. Lowered reaction time and increased sluggishness make it more likely that women in the paramenstrum will be caught during their misconduct.

Lowered levels of estrogen and progesterone during the paramen-stral week may affect women's behavior, but there are many links between the cause and its effect. Changes in the level of the female sex hormones can hardly be the direct cause of the reported incidence of children's illnesses normally associated with the paramenstrum. Dalton speculates that during the paramenstrum a mother loses the tolerance needed to look after a sick child. Her patience is short and she will more readily pick up the phone and call the doctor or bring the child to the doctor's office. During the other phases of the cycle, presumably, her patience is more enduring and she is less likely to report a minor illness.†

* I might add that in the end I canceled the scheduled surgery and changed gynecologists.
† Dalton suggests one other possible cause-and-effect relationship in this instance. Higher levels of paramenstral tension may create stresses in a child which can lead to the development of a minor illness.

The most alarming statistic of paramenstral behavior is that 50 percent of the women who attempt or complete suicidal acts are in this phase of cycle. Whatever the complex relationship between emotional, environmental, and physiological factors contributing to this situation, any changes in hormone level must be carefully scrutinized since this is the one aspect of the web that can most easily be modified.

Reviewing the literature on the relationship between suicide and time of cycle, Wetzel and McClure[13] found that the methods used in the various studies were so markedly different from one another that a compilation or comparison of findings was impossible.

The relationship between suicidal behavior and time of menstrual cycle will remain unclear until the designs of the experiments themselves are improved. Obviously, should future research confirm this relationship, work on the nature of hormone output must become a priority for public health research so that hormone levels can be modified for those people who show a sensitivity to hormonal variation.

The fact that the physiological changes of the paramenstral phase appear to have some effect on woman's behavior (physical and emotional resistance to stress appears to lower, and the body and spirit have more difficulty coping at this phase than at others) describes the trend of the research cited above but tells us nothing about the contribution of environmental stresses to the coping mechanism. These changes, after all, conform all too well with the social evaluation that menstruation is a debilitating experience and a cornerstone of female inferiority.

Relatively little research has been done on all this. So far, there is no foundation from which to understand the link between the internal changes of the hormone cycle and the external demands of the menstrual taboo. For example, we don't know the extent to which the taboo exacerbates the physical changes that occur during the paramenstrum or the extent to which the beliefs underlying the taboo actually cause these problems.

I recently spoke with a young woman who had suffered from premenstrual depression since her teen years. She knew that the depressions occurred before menstruation but, initially, she believed that this was a unique and peculiar problem. After a couple of years she learned that many other women suffer with premenstrual depression. When she had learned that she was not alone—that she was not afflicted with a cosmic punishment—her sense of relief was enormous.

The depression had not entirely disappeared, but its effect had decreased dramatically. While she would like to be free from the remaining depression, she no longer is frightened by her feelings. Furthermore, the suicidal feelings which used to accompany her monthly depressions have completely disappeared. She now knows that the depression will end as menstrual flow begins, and her ability to endure has strengthened.

Not long after this discussion took place I had the opportunity to accompany a friend who was going for a voice lesson. Midway through her class, the maestro beckoned her and whispered in her ear. She turned to me and said he had asked if she was menstruating. (In fact she was due to begin the next day.) When asked why he posed this question, the coach replied that most singers lose some muscle control during menstruation and that he could hear the loss in the quality of voice production. His wife, herself a concert singer, was also present and told us that most singers schedule their performance outside the menstrual interval for this reason.

I have told these stories to other women in the course of Know Your Body classes at the Women's Health Forum in New York. On several occasions, individual women became incensed after hearing them. How dare I suggest that menstruation might have any effect on behavior or that a menstrual difficulty might have to be *endured* (or endured until further research alleviates the problem)? No amount of discussion of the other aspects of the cycle, the times of high self-esteem and solid feelings of competition, had the slightest effect on the anger of these women. Menstruation, they seemed to believe, ought not to exist in any of its manifestations. The body (or more exactly, woman's body) should not have *any* specific effect on woman's feelings or outlook. Such vehemence directed toward denial of the menstrual cycle is understandable. Nonetheless, it is another manifestation of the legacy of the taboo and another way in which women accept that taboo and fight their own bodies and feelings rather than learning from one another the actual nature of menstruation.

Anger, embarrassment, or avoidance are all ways of dealing with the cycle's influence on behavior. They are also ways of rendering these influences an assault, rather than understanding them and then going on to look at the ways in which environment plays its important role.

Some of the relationships between feeling, behavior, and time of cycle seem particularly trivial, yet they contribute to the ways in which a woman evaluates herself in the world of other people. For example, we have seen that just prior to menstruation a woman's feelings of self-esteem may be at their lowest point, while at ovulation she feels a high degree of self-confidence. Just before menstruation, a look in the mirror is likely to show limp hair, sallow skin, and a flare-up of adolescent acne—all seen through puffy eyes.

The menstrual uglies . . . a few days before menstruation many women look somewhat more tired; the glowing edge of a healthy look wanes. In most cases the alteration in appearance is very slight, but many times the *feeling* of loss of looks is intense. Women often become anxious at the slightest loss of attractiveness (since looks are our most widely acknowledged asset) and see it for more than it is. The menstrual uglies provide a particularly clear example of the way in which a minor aspect of the premenstrual phase becomes more substantial because of the social evaluation of the female role.

Men, of course, may be considered attractive because of good looks or because they are clever, rich, learned, or accomplished. Women are said to be attractive when they are physically attractive—and the measure of this is sexual drawing power. To further complicate the image of the sexually attractive woman, she must appear to be within the age range dictated by menstruation (she must have the potential for being a danger to man), but she must not show any physical sign that menstruation or cyclicity exists.

The cultural belief that menstruation is a fall from feminine grace is felt by women most strongly at the time when menstrual flow is expected. Most women are virtually bound to feel less attractive at this phase of the cycle. When a small loss of attractiveness actually occurs just before flow it triggers underlying convictions that we are, by nature, unappealing during menstruation.

At the coming of the menstrual phase of the cycle, a woman is approaching that point at which men consider her the gravest threat. Ideals of feminine beauty vary according to the culture, but the belief that menstruating woman is corrupt and unclean is universal, and women begin to take special precautions at the time of menstruation. Throughout Latin America, for example, women do not eat acid fruits or drink their juice; in Europe, women refrain from preparing certain foods; Brahmin women of India are forbidden to cook *any* food; and in Burma some foods must not be touched for fear they will turn sour.

Different religious traditions may develop varied ideals of femininity, but many religions consider menstruating woman unclean and demand that she keep outside the religious society until she is "safe" again.

> We command the woman in her period not enter the temple nor to sacrifice to the gods *uabilca* and if they should enter let them be punished.[14]

> It may be added that, of comparatively recent times, Catholic theologians have regarded intercourse during menstruation as a sin. Icard points out that some Catholic theologians have declared that intercourse during menstruation, if not a mortal sin, is at least a venial sin. Sanchez, I may remark, states that many theologians consider it a mortal sin to seek intercourse during menstruation.[15]

> And if a woman have an issue, and her issue in her flesh be blood, she shall be put apart seven days and whosoever toucheth her shall be unclean until the even.
> And if any man lie with her at all, and her flowers be upon him, he shall be unclean seven days; and all the bed whereon he lieth shall be unclean.
> But even if she be cleansed of her issue, then she shall number to herself seven days, and after that she shall be clean.
> —Leviticus XV:19;24;28.

> They ask thee concerning women's courses. Say: They are a hurt and a pollution. —The Koran S. II. 222.

The Incas, of course, are no more, and the present-day Catholic Church no longer maintains any religious proscriptions on menstruating women. However, among Orthodox Jews and Christian sects that take the Bible as a literal guide to life, the teachings of Leviticus still stand as law.

Jewish women are not permitted to pray in the temple during the menstrual period, Brahmin women of India are not permitted to any holy place while they menstruate, and the women of Islam are not permitted to recite the daily prayers or to enter a mosque while menstruating. Among members of the Nation of Islam (frequently called Black Muslims), women are not permitted to say their daily prayers but are permitted to enter the temple.* However, they do not actively participate in prayer at the temple until menstruation, the time of cleansing, has stopped.

---

* In the East, the mosque is the holy place for followers of Islam. Followers of the Hon. Elijah Mohammed consider the temple a place of teaching; it therefore serves many purposes besides that of a place in which to pray.

Karen Paige speculated that the ways in which women experience menstruation would be influenced by the concepts present in the religions they practice.[16] She suspected that the particular qualities of the taboo transmitted through religious training would have particular effects on women, so she prepared a set of questions that would elicit general information about the level of physical and emotional health of each woman studied. She also solicited information about attitudes toward femininity. These were divided into three categories: feelings about family and motherhood; sexual experience; and acceptance of the menstrual taboo. The subjects were 298 unmarried college students: 54 were Jewish, 181 Protestant, and 63 Catholic.

Paige found that among Jewish women, those most likely to have difficulties with menstruation were the women who accepted the ban on sexual intercourse during menstruation. Among the Catholic women, those who accepted the belief with which they were raised (that it is woman's lot to suffer) also believed that menstrual distress is a fact of woman's life. They *expected* to have problems with menstruation. Furthermore, Paige states that the more fully these women lived out the feminine role ideal with which they were brought up, the *more frequent* were their premenstrual problems.* Those who were married, had children, and had no substantial goal outside the home had the most severe menstrual difficulty. Paige found no particular pattern of menstrual experience among the Protestant women in her study, a fact she attributes to a failure to subdivide the subjects according to the various Protestant sects.

This study strongly indicates that women who have accepted the menstrual taboo, and the concept of femininity it describes, are most likely to have problems with the experience of menstruation.† She concludes:

> I have come to believe that the "raging hormones" theory of menstrual distress simply isn't adequate. Nor do I agree with the "raging-neurosis" theory, which argues that women who have menstrual symptoms are merely whining neurotics, who need only a kind of pat on the head to cure their problems.
>
> We must instead consider the problem from the perspective of

* These findings may be compared with those of Bart discussed in the following chapter (pp. 204–6) which show that severe menopausal depression parallels the most avid acceptance of the conventional super-mother identification.
† This is the exact opposite of the shaman's view that menstrual problems are *caused* by refusal to adopt the constraints of the taboo.

women's subordinate social position, and of the cultural ideology that so narrowly defines the behaviors that are appropriately "feminine." Women have perfectly good reasons to react emotionally to reproductive events. . . . Her reproductive abilities define her femininity; other routes to success are only second best in this society.[17]

Somewhere between the denial of the menstrual cycle and its bearing on behavior and the overzealous acceptance of only the negative aspects of cyclic variation rests a balanced assessment of the ways in which the cycle of menstruation (as well as that of menopause) shapes woman's experience. The taboo and its subsequent prejudices form a straitjacket, constricting emotional and intellectual growth. If the flight from taboo leads to the denial of the menstrual cycle, it is as constricting as docile acceptance.

As long as women run from the reality of the menstrual cycle, we are refusing to know ourselves and are accepting an external definition of ourselves. Harding says:

> . . . Life may present a woman with an opportunity for work or for a spiritual adventure for which she has long waited. If the moon is favorable, she is able to take the step which will lead her out into a freer life of greater opportunity, but if the moon is not favorable she may see her longed-for chance slip by and be unable to do anything effective to seize it. . . . It requires an act of devotion deeper than at first seemed necessary, if a woman is to live her life in harmony with the rhythm of her own nature.
>
> Yet when she recognizes that this all-powerful fate is *not* wielded by some outside power, by an inaccessible deity of the moon, but is instead the expression of the essential nature of her own being, she will feel very differently about it. For the rhythmic life within her is determinant of her own life, while her conscious wishes and impulses do not necessarily coincide with her deepest needs. . . .
>
> No human being is wise enough to know from his past experience what course his life should take in the future. . . . Consciously he can only look forward in complete blindness to the future. But his future is surely determined by his own nature. For woman, at all events, the moon "goddess," that is, the feminine principle within her, plays a hand and she usually holds the trump cards.[18]

It is impossible for women at this particular moment fully to understand what it means when Harding says the moon goddess usually holds the trump cards. We cannot know because we have only just begun to consider the possibility that such a spirit resides within us.

To confront this spirit, and learn the many faces of the reality of the menstrual cycle, we must break through defenses which protect us from admitting that we are considered cursed. These defenses also protect us from feeling menstrual shame. Perhaps we will first have to do battle with this feeling before there is freedom to consider the many other feelings that exist.

The menstrual taboo has a far greater control over the destiny of women than does the spirit of the moon goddess. She does not control woman's destiny but rather gives it a certain conformation. The cyclic nature of menstruating woman is only a part of the nature of woman—yet the taboo has defined the entire nature of female existence.

From drug company to advertising agency, from gynecologist to patient . . . The following pictures and slogans were created to help gynecologists identify "women's complaints" and to help them assume the correct pose when prescribing treatment. All of the advertisements (portions of which are deleted here) originally appeared in medical journals.

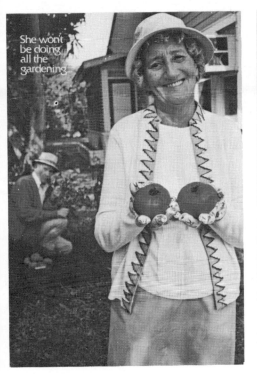

She won't be doing all the gardening...

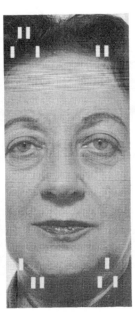

but she can still grow some of the juiciest tomatoes in the neighborhood

For many elderly, estrogen deficient women, activities that once were simple may now be too much.

Predictability... proven with time. The enduring value of Miltown.

(meprobamate) 400 mg tablets

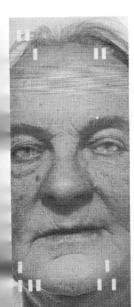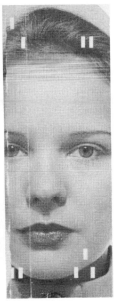

With proper patient selection, these are the cases you can expect to respond...

Patients with somatic complaints, when anxiety and tension are present:
as an adjunct, anticipate response in...
· tension headache
· anxiety and tension accompanying organic disease
· behavioral and social adjustments

Geriatric patients:
anticipate response in...
· senile agitation, restlessness, irritability
· sleep disturbances

Preoperative or pre-hospitalized patients:
as an adjunct, anticipate response in...
· apprehension prior to hospitalization or surgery

WALLACE PHARMACEUTICALS Cranbury, N.J. 08512

Please see following page for brief summary of prescribing information.

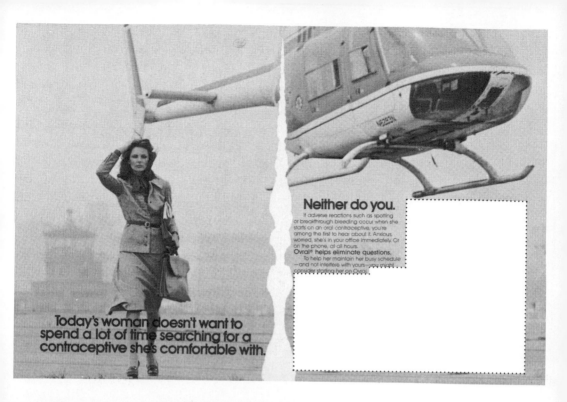

Today's woman doesn't want to spend a lot of time searching for a contraceptive she's comfortable with.

Neither do you.

If adverse reactions such as spotting or breakthrough bleeding occur when she starts on an oral contraceptive, you're among the first to hear about it. Anxious, worried, she's in your office immediately. Or on the phone, at all hours.

Ovral® helps eliminate questions.

To help her maintain her busy schedule —and not interfere with yours—you might consider starting her on Ovral.

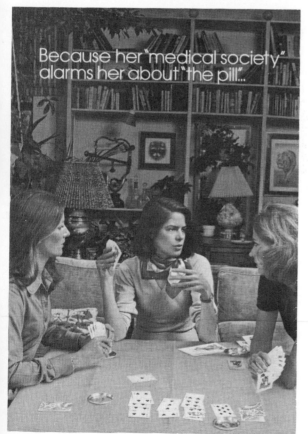

Because her "medical society" alarms her about "the pill"...

and because she runs to you for her answer

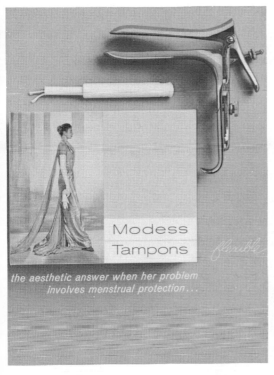
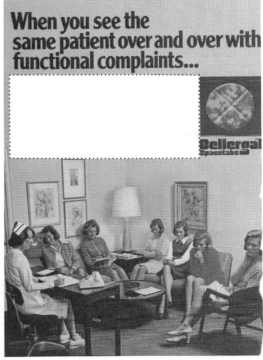
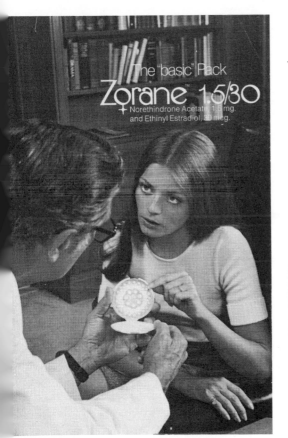
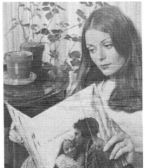

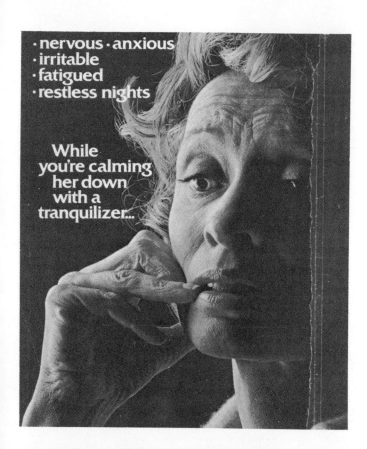
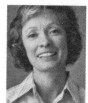
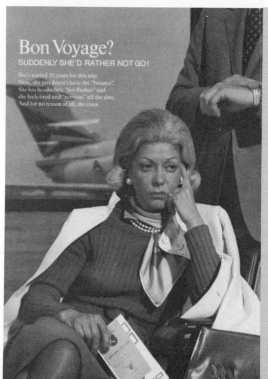

9

Unveiled
and Invisible

Not long after her thirtieth birthday a woman begins searching the mirror for signs of age. Each one sighted is carefully studied. These moments in which the glance lingers are tender, as though one had always longed to see what getting old would look like. The feeling is sweet because what is seen is only a preview.

A few years pass and looking in the mirror becomes a game of darts. The eyes travel on beams of light directly to the signs of age, land for a split second, and flick away. We see ourselves ageing only in these fragmented seconds. The remainder of our time is spent looking at the blurred and generalized image.

Women in this society don't want to get old for many reasons. We do not want to face the implications of ageing and therefore refuse to face the image of ourselves as having aged. But however skilled a woman becomes at the game of mirror darts, a moment comes when she *knows* she has aged. This is the moment of menopause.

Contrary to popular belief, menopause and ageing are not dreadful diseases or conditions. In part, these beliefs are a result of rather wild rumors about the troubles of menopause, and in part they are a realistic reflection of the social position of older women in our society.

In the menstrual survey, I asked if there was anything women wanted to know about menopause. The overwhelming majority made no response to this question at all. A few replied that they had never thought about it, but now that it was mentioned, they had better

begin to learn what it is. Two women who did wonder about menopause wrote:

Is it true that women go crazy while going through menopause?

(ANON, *age seventeen*)

*I'd like to know what to expect from menopause. I tend to be nervous
and edgy now. . . . I worry about going crazy or losing all control
when I reach menopause. I am twenty-one now, so I'll just have to
wait and see.* (D.G.)

Millions of women have heard stories about menopause but don't
know about the realities of the experience. Like the woman quoted
above, they will have thirty years or more in which to wait and see,
and wait and worry, and wait and expect the worst. In each passing
year they are likely to become more (not less) convinced that menopause is a horror because unexamined anxiety is likely to feed itself,
not cure itself.

For men, menopause is, of course, not an emotionally loaded issue;
in many cases they consider the menopausal woman a rather comic
figure. She is pictured with a red face, erratic moods, and the ultimate
parcel of female troubles. They may patronize her and pity her sad
condition, or wonder how they can aid the poor creature who is about
to pass through a "profound life crisis."

Prompted perhaps by observing these male attitudes, women have
begun to ask about the existence of a male menopause. The desire to
find a male equivalent to menopause is understandable. If men experienced menopause, we rightfully suspect that it would be given
greater respect, subjected to more basic research, and would gain
more credibility.

A distinction must be made here between menopause and the
climacteric. Menopause refers *only* to the cessation of menstruation,
the discreet changes in sex hormones which underlie it, and the
termination of fertility. Menopause occurs over a relatively brief
period of a year or two, during which highly specific biological
changes occur. While menopause functions as an event symbolic of
ageing, it is fundamentally a biological event.

The *climacteric* describes the transition made during a period of
fifteen to twenty years between the biological state of middle age and
that of older age (roughly spanning the period between one's mid-
forties and mid-sixties). Climacteric changes, therefore, may be observed in all bodily tissue and body systems in members of both sexes.

Within the context of the climacteric, menopause is only one event taking place in the female body.

Men do not experience menopause. There is no clear-cut period during which the male sex hormones drop in production and realign at a new, lower level. There are, therefore, no male symptoms which are the by-products of profound hormonal readjustment. (Men, of course, retain fertility throughout their lives.) Males do not experience a biological event that symbolizes the arrival of age, but they do most certainly experience climacteric changes, among which is the decrease in potency, along with the ageing process of tissues and bodily systems that affects every part of the body.

> With advancing years, the woman faces a moment when giving up her productive maternity will occur as irrevocably and unmistakenly as the beginning was once signaled at menarche. But the male's loss of potential paternity, like the diminution of his potency, is gradual, indefinite, reversible. It has neither the quality of a single devastating event, which is the way women often experience menopause, nor the possibility of a peaceful acceptance of a consummated step in life, which is also possible to women. He keeps the rewards and the psychological hazards that go with a less punctuated ageing process.[1]

During their middle years, men, of course, confront changes in their potency and changes in their placement in the job market. A man no longer has his entire future giving promise of grander things to come and is likely now to re-evaluate the success he has or has not achieved. He will also become increasingly aware of the presence of younger people who are interested in having his job in their future. It is generally understood that a man will "weather" his crises and continue to command respect. He will reap the rewards still available—of which there are many.

Women often feel that menopause is a black cloud hovering overhead. This cloud begins to take form during the years of fertility in which women are taught the myths of the fertile goddess and transcendent madonna. During the fertile years, the mirror image has an added glow because it partakes of this mythic aura. When the first signs of ageing are sighted, their existence makes the glow even more precious by comparison. But the woman looking into the mirror doesn't realize that the glowing image exists only because she has accepted a myth which *includes* the horror of age. The black cloud is made of all that will be lost when age comes, and its specter helps to make women seize on the myths of the fertile woman while they can. All are convinced that later a woman will be riddled with physical problems, will lose her fertility and be cast aside. After all, what makes the first sighting of age a tender moment is the reassurance that it has not yet come, that one is still young enough to reap the rewards given to the young and fertile woman.

Because we are a people with a horror of ageing and dread of death, it is not surprising that youth is perceived as the glittering time of life and age as tarnished. The idolization of youth, a logical extension of these fears, has taken on an independent veracity; we have come to believe that youth is intrinsically marvelous. Obviously, when youth is considered a blessing, the end of youth by definition is a dreadful event. Attitudes toward menstruation and menopause mirror this pattern of reasoning.

Menopause is feared because it is associated with being old. A "separate" truth emerges in which the nubile woman is considered blessed (even though her blessing includes the curse). The more avidly one embraces the belief that motherhood is holy and fertility golden, the greater the conviction that menopause is the corrosive end to all that is desirable and worthwhile.

Once menopause is identified as the end to the best time of life, it naturally looms as a life crisis and its impending occurrence exerts formidable pressures on younger women. These fears and pressures convince women that they had better accept the definitions of femininity which accompany the equation of youth and fertility with blessing, since these appear to be the only rewards available and they are rewards with a very limited timetable.

Fifty or sixty years ago, the picture of a glowing feminine fertility and a dreary, painful menopause may have been a terrible burden for many women; but menopause was in all probability an event that took place shortly before one's death.* Today, with a quarter century of life to follow, this two-sided image is not supportable at all. If young women put all their attention and energy toward the prevailing image of femininity, they are sentencing themselves to twenty-five years of partial life. If women do not do this, then the years of menopause and post-menopause will not represent the darkness after the golden dawn, for they will not (internally at least) be appreciably different from the years before.†

---

* At the turn of this century, menopause occurred during a woman's forties; her life expectancy was forty-nine years.

† Implied in this change of attitude, of course, is the end to the "privilege" now associated with being a fertile young woman. These privileges, we cannot forget, are paid for with the agreement that they will be lost at the coming of menopause.

Today the average woman in America has menopause at the age of fifty and a life expectancy of seventy-five years; she can expect to live a quarter of a century past the time of menopause. Women who are sharing this experience now grew up in an era when the definition of the female role accepted by the majority of women—willingly or reluctantly—centered on fertility and motherhood.*

In the seventies, despite the heightened expectations of women and the opportunities which have, to some extent, increased, the status and roles of menopausal and postmenopausal women are still being overlooked. When menopause *is* discussed, it is in the socially acceptable context of its physiological problems. A woman's position in society, however, is less openly considered, and when it is discussed it is usually in isolation. There is, for example, a separate movement called Older Women's Liberation, as though there were two separate female sexes divided by age.†

Older women have been forced into a somewhat separatist movement because they have been ignored by those who are younger. Most young women—and men—who are older but not yet of an age where menopause is imminent prefer to ignore the issue of menopause and ageing. For most of us these issues are unsettling and until the passage of time forces us, we would rather ignore them altogether.

What is known about the experience of menopause apart from its black image? What, if any, truth is there in the stories of horror? Is it a crisis that is fearful, or is it an experience in life like all the others with particular qualities, its own advantages and liabilities?

Menopause has occurred when twelve consecutive months have passed without menstruation. The experience bears many physiological and emotional similarities to puberty: both are times of hormone realignment and physical upheaval, and both may result in the production of physical or emotional symptoms. Apart from the actual ages at which these experiences occur, one difference between them is crucial. Puberty is the time when a girl enters womanhood (signaled by the start of menstrual cycles and fertility), while menopause is considered the end to womanhood (signaled by the loss of menstrua-

---

* As recently as the 1950s, a woman who did not wear a wedding band or push a baby carriage was hardly considered a woman at all. This makes the phenomenon of fifties nostalgia seem particularly bizarre. Never mind the clothes, music, or fancy steps, the mental baggage women lugged around is best buried in cultural history; *it* doesn't get more attractive with the passing of time.

† Every group of women naturally has particular problems and special interests. However, there are no separate movements such as single women's liberation, mother's liberation, or teen-age women's liberation. We witness only O.W.L.

tion and fertility). The meaning attached to each aspect of hormonal change, as well as the meaning attached to any symptoms which develop, is charged with the different values society attaches to each time of life.

The young woman is subjected to an intensive social campaign in which she must begin at once to act as a feminine creature. Social education is stressed and the changes in her hormones are almost completely ignored. Thirty or forty years pass in which recurrent cycles of hormone change have formed the substrata of woman's experience. During these years the litany is sung and repeated: you are your reproductive functions; you are the madonna and the whore. Menopause occurs, and women will never again experience the monthly flow of blood or the monthly cycles of hormonal change. As soon as the bleeding ends, the menstrual taboo stops and the values attached to womanhood are no more.

The menopausal woman has had her social education. Within its framework her soul is now of little importance because fertility and "dangerous" menstruation no longer form part of her being. Her body is no longer unclean, but it no longer serves its most "important" function—that of giving form to fertility. This body, however, "lingers" on and what remains becomes the focus of anxious attention.

Menopause—Its Relationship to Behavior

The shaman paves the way for the "critical" event. He reminds women at every opportunity that menopause looms in their future, and he reminds them that it is a physical crisis. A woman must remember that fertility is femininity and that when it begins to wane, and when it finally ends, she will be beset by all sorts of problems.

> . . . Women are told, in their early thirties, that their ills are due to the approach of the menopause. In their forties, the ills are blamed on the existence of the menopause. Then the menopause actually takes place. And even should it go very smoothly, any illnesses that come later are blamed on the fact that the menopause is past. It almost seems as if, after a woman reaches adulthood, her whole life is made to revolve around this single event.[2]

Departing from the world of magic and divinity, the psychologists Neugarten and Kraines undertook a study to find out what symptoms are common to women of different age groups.[3] These researchers were among the first to seek information directly from women about what women actually experience. Just what *do* women feel during menopause? How does this differ from the way women feel at other stages of life?

To get the answer to these questions, the investigators polled 460 women. The women were divided into five groups—the youngest in their adolescence, the oldest sixty-four. Each group represented an age category, but the women between ages forty-four and fifty-five were divided into two separate groups—those who were either pre- or postmenopausal and those who were in the midst of menopause. Each group reported their physical and emotional symptoms.

In analyzing their results, Neugarten and Kraines noted that adolescents and menopausal women reported the largest number of symptoms. *Postmenopausal women reported the smallest number of symptoms.* Apparently menopause does not cause such havoc that women's health is ruined for the remainder of their lives. On the contrary, after menopause women have the easiest time in terms of physical and emotional symptomology.

Among the adolescents studied, "psychological" symptoms (tension, for example) were most common, while the menopausal women generally suffered with physical problems (hot flushes, for example). Similar physiological changes underlie the production of adolescent and menopausal symptomology, but the kind of symptoms experienced mirror the social evaluation of each stage—adolescence is seen as a psychological event of great proportions, while menopause is alleged to be a grave physical crisis. "These findings suggest . . . that it is the increased production of sex hormones during adolescence (signaled by the first menses) and the decreased production of estrogen during the climacterum (signaled by the menopause) that are primary in producing heightened sensitivity to and increased frequency of reported symptoms."[*4] There were four categories in which menopausal women reported a greater incidence of symptoms that might be called psychological. These were headache, irritability and nervousness, feeling blue, and feelings of suffocation. (The last-named symptom is a common corollary to hot flushes.) The authors believe that, "Because of her experience and maturity . . . [menopausal woman] has learned to cope more effectively at the psychological level with biological change and biological stress than has the adolescent."[5]

---

[*] The symptoms of women in the 44–55-year-old group were greater among the menopausal women than those who were pre- or postmenopausal. Age was not the symptom-producing factor.

Observing the claim that menopause is a time when otherwise healthy women experience many distressing physical symptoms but that few have chosen to verify this hypothesis, Sonja M. McKinlay and Margot Jefferys (working in the area of medical sociology) published the results of a study conducted in London in the years 1964–65.[6]

In their study, McKinlay and Jefferys polled 638 women between the ages of forty-five and fifty-four by means of a questionnaire sent out in the mail. They divided the respondents into eleven categories according to their menstrual or menopausal status, which ranged from women who were menstruating "regularly" to those who had not had a menstrual period in more than nine years. The symptoms studied were hot flushes, night sweats, headache, dizzy spells, palpitations, sleeplessness, depression, and weight gain.

The authors report that from 30 to 50 percent of the women experienced dizziness, palpitations, insomnia, depression, headache, and weight gain, and that if one symptom were observed usually several went together. The frequency with which these symptoms was reported did not vary greatly from one subgroup to the next, although there was an increase between the "regular" and "irregular" menstruation groups. There was no one peak at which these symptom clusters appeared and no one point at which the frequency of discomfort diminished. These facts led the investigators to conclude that such symptoms are not directly related to the menopause.

Almost one half (48.5 percent) of the women reported hot flushes and half of this group (or almost 25 percent of the total) said the flushes were acutely uncomfortable. Another 20.5 percent of the women who had flushes stated that, while they did not suffer physical distress, they had felt embarrassed. (Less than one in five of the women with flushes had consulted a physician for relief of symptoms.) For women who still had regular menstrual experiences, hot flushes rarely occurred, while four out of five menopausal women experienced them. Some degree of flushing continued throughout the postmenopausal subgroups, tapering off in the group who had their last flow more than nine years before. Hot flushes, then, are clearly directly related to menopause—a fact which other investigators support.

Sonja McKinlay and John B. McKinlay put out an annotated bibliography of ninety-four papers published during the past thirty years which deal with menopause.[7] A careful review of the methods used by the various researchers, as well as their findings, led the

McKinlays to suggest a list of research questions in need of answers. This list includes the need for a definition of the menopausal syndrome that accurately reflects women's experience, as well as a need to distinguish between symptoms of menopause and those of the postmenopause. Thus far we can only be sure that hot flushes are clearly related to the experience of menopause and that, in most cases, it seems that estrogen replacement therapy successfully alleviates this symptom.

As a young woman in puberty, the female is left to cope as best she can. Older women have learned (at whatever cost) to cope more effectively and, according to the study done by Neugarten and Kraines, can look forward to a healthier period of life in their postmenopause. Women are aided in their coping by the knowledge that menopause is a temporary state. Why then is menopause a bugaboo; why do women continue to fear that they will lose their minds and become physical wrecks?

One explanation, of course, is the lack of research. While physicians put a great deal of emphasis on changes in menstrual experience in the years just before the expected onset of menopause (and in so doing create an atmosphere of anxiety), they do little to learn the nature of specifically menopausal symptoms and the expected duration of any such symptoms.

The reports of physicians based on their experience in clinical practice (which is hardly the most authoritative form of information on the experience of the overall population) indicate that only 10 percent of menopausal women experience symptoms so severe that they are incapacitated. It is possible that the fear of a terrible menopause is predicated on the rumors about the experience of this minority. In the absence of concrete information and in the presence of medically induced anxiety, it is not surprising that the reports of the worst experiences have taken precedence over the commonplace but less dramatic experience of the majority.

We have already learned that women who suffer so severely at menopause are, in general, those whose hormone supply has dramatically declined. This informs us of the physiological reality but tells us little about women's fear of their future menopausal experience. After all, no one can successfully predict which women will experience a slow tapering-off in hormone production and which women the symptom-producing sharp drop-off. Anxiety feeds on uncertainty. If we examine the emotional experience of the small group within the minority with severe symptoms who suffer psychic distress of high degree, we may gain insight into the dark image so many women fear will be their future selves.

The sociologist Pauline Bart studied the phenomenon of middle-aged depression occurring during the interval in which menopause may be expected to appear (between the ages of forty and fifty-nine).[8] She examined case histories of 533 women who were hospitalized for the first time between the ages of forty and fifty-nine. Of these women, almost one half had been institutionalized for depression (ranging from neurotic to psychotic); the remainder had been diagnosed as suffering from one or another functional disability (schizophrenia, for example). After comparing these records, Bart concluded:

> Women who have overprotective or overinvolved relationships with their children are more likely to suffer depression in their postparental period than women who do not have such relationships. Housewives have a higher rate of depression than working women. . . . Not only do housewives have more opportunity than working women to invest themselves completely in their children, but the housewife role is cut down once there are fewer people for whom to shop, cook and clean.
>
> Middle-class housewives have a higher rate of depression than working-class housewives, and those housewives who have overprotective relationships with their children suffer the highest rate of depression of all when the children leave home.[9]

Among the 10 percent of women who suffer severe menopausal distress, a small number develop depressions that are incapacitating. We are talking about a very small percentage of women whose experience does not reflect the common experience of their age mates, but their experience is nonetheless instructive.

During adolescence, women are taught that to be feminine they must be both wife and mother—the more enthusiastically these roles are embraced, the greater their rewards will be. During the fertile years the shaman repeatedly tells women that any disorder with menstruation, any difficulty or pain, is the result of her failure to be enthusiastic about this role. And during the time of menopause, the women who are walking along the correct path, who have subscribed to the menstrual taboo and carry out the allotted actions, are likely to be its primary casualties.*

To some still unknown degree, the likelihood of suffering from a

---

* This conclusion from Bart's research parallels that found by Paige and reported in the preceding chapter: women who most actively support the menstrual taboo suffer the greatest amount of difficulty with menstruation.

depression of this intensity depends on the severity of hormone loss. We know, for example, that depression is a symptom common to many women who have the menopausal syndrome. It may be that when a woman suffers from an extreme case of menopausal syndrome and when the role she plays is the one defined by Bart above, the depression brought by hormonal changes is dreadfully intensified.

We might expect that the rate of hormone decline (and the degree of symptom formation produced accordingly) would occur uniformly, with little regard for race, religion, or creed, and that the same would hold true for symptoms experienced. Bart has shown, however, that in serious cases of middle-aged depression among women, this is not the case: "When ethnic groups are compared, Jews have the highest rate of depression, Anglos an intermediate rate, and blacks the lowest rate."[10]

According to this study, then, the Jewish mother shows the highest incidence of middle-aged depression. (Jewish women whose mothers were born in the U.S. showed a rate of depression midway between that of Jewish women whose mothers were born abroad and Anglo women.) Traditionally, she focuses on her family's life intensely and has no well-defined role once the family leaves home. And traditionally, she has been the object of humor because she goes on caring intensely when her family no longer wants or needs her attention.

> It is very easy to make fun of these women, to ridicule their pride in their children and concern for their well-being. But it is no mark of real progress to substitute Molly Goldberg for Stepin Fetchitt as a stock comedy figure. These women are as much casualties of our culture as the children in Harlem whose I.Q.s decline with each additional year they spend in school.[11]

Bart offers four hypotheses to explain the lower incidence of middle-aged depression among black women:

> The patterns of black female-role behavior rarely result in depression in middle age. Often, the "granny" or "aunty" lives with the family and cares for the children while the children's mother works; thus, the older woman suffers no maternal role loss. Second since black women traditionally work, they are less likely to develop the extreme identification, the vicarious living through their children that is characteristic of Jewish mothers. In addition, there is no puritanical idea in black culture equivalent to that in Anglo and Jewish cultures, that sex is evil and primarily for reproductive purposes. . . .
> Of course, one cannot entirely overlook the possibility that the low black depression rate simply reflects the black communities' unwilling-

ness to hospitalize depressed black women. Depressives are not likely to come to the attention of the police unless they attempt suicide.[12]

Bart did another study in which she reviewed anthropological accounts of the status of women in 150 cultures. She found that while the specific attributes and ideals of feminine behavior varied widely, one generalization was applicable to all cultures: whatever the role of women during the fertile years, it is *reversed* at menopause. Following are three specific cases I found in my research which support her findings. Margaret Mead observes:

> Where reproductivity has been regarded as somewhat impure and ceremonially disqualifying—as in Bali—the post-menopausal woman and the virgin girl work together at ceremonies in which women of childbearing age are debarred. Where modesty of speech and action is enjoined on women, such behavior may no longer be asked from the older woman, who may use obscene language as freely or more freely than any man.[13]

M. J. Levy comments:

> The *lao-nien* stage was often an unusual one for women. It was often a stage in which a woman was released from male domination. The ancient formula held that as a child she was subject to her father, as a woman to her husband, and as a widow to her son. . . . By the time her sons were mature and she was widowed, a Chinese woman was likely to be a *lao-nien*. . . . Hers was almost the only situation in which a woman could really shake off male domination and assume domination over males without incurring definite social disapproval. Moreover, any attempt to "put her in her place," save in extreme cases, would probably have been socially disapproved.[14]

and in Clara Thompson's view:

> By far the greatest hazards of the menopause are psychogenical or culturally induced, and these are not so simply dispelled by a few pills. A psychiatrist working in China reported to me that she had never seen a menopausal psychosis in a Chinese woman. This she attributed to the fact that in China the older woman has a secure and coveted position.[15]

None of these examples provides us with a model of a society in which women live a more privileged life than we. Balinese or pre-revolutionary Chinese cultures created environments in which during her fertile years a woman's life was limited and impoverished by the proscriptions of the menstrual taboo and her low status—only *after* menopause does this improve. However, the example of these cultures demonstrates that it is the cultural attitudes toward older women, not the biological realities of menopause, that are responsible for the meaning attached to menopause and ageing. In some cases, these attitudes are also responsible for the kinds of symptoms that develop.

We can point to any culture in which menopausal women have a higher status as an example of the relativity of roles granted to women. There is nothing about menopause which in itself leads to the low status of the postmenopausal woman in the United States. Menopause (for at least 90 percent of women) does not in itself cause debilitation, nor does it so weaken women that they may not function as powerful members of the community. Our cultural inheritance has dictated that woman is valued and valuable *only* as long as she can reproduce. " 'Woman,' Virchow is reported to have said, 'is a pair of ovaries with a human being attached; whereas man is a human being furnished with a pair of testes.' "[16]

In the early part of the twentieth century, Dr. Ploss and the Bartleses compiled a three-volume work which attempted to cover every aspect of female life as observed by men. Their attitudes toward women, as indicated by the quotation above, still flourish today. There is a popular saying among gynecologists that there is no ovary so healthy that it is not better removed, and no testes so diseased they should not be left intact.

In 1715, The Faithful Eckharth gave us this image of a young woman's beauty and its destruction with the passage of time:

> Just as in young women, so long as their blooming takes its orderly course all is in full flower and motion, so with those women who have lost their bloom all spirit and briskness decline. The color which excites love changes to a faded paleness, the once tense muscles and flesh-covered fibres become slack, and wrinkles take the place of the former smoothness, and beauty; indeed, the whole form is altered so that when one compares the present figure with the earlier beauty, it is difficult to find any likeness. The eyes which used to dart hither and thither, like those of falcons, become dull and glazed. The lovely cheeks fall in, the ruby lips become plum color, brown and dull, the well-grown spine curves and bends and with it the erect neck, the beautiful skin becomes yellowish; the flesh disappears from those pretty hands and feet. In fine, all that a lover once held beautiful, is now repulsive to him and arouses in him disgust and horror of uncomeliness.[17]

All the suppressed fear and envy of woman which men feel during her fertile years is unleashed in the form of mockery or outright hatred.

Whatever else contributed to Eckharth's perceptions, his are the revelations of a faithless lover. He is now free from his terror of the fertile woman and can safely vent his rage. Because she no longer has the power to make him afraid, she no longer has the potential to harm him.

A look through any current medical journal will provide plenty of visual evidence that menopausal woman continues to be perceived as a physical wreck. In these periodicals the middle-aged men are always distinguished-looking, but the women are beset by wrinkles, stringy hair, and dull eyes.

The higher status given to men is matched by their egotism. They, of course, become distinguished with the passing years; whatever alterations in the appearance age brings are additions, not subtractions. Even if a woman should overcome incredible "obstacles" and maintain her beauty throughout her years, she is still seen as no match for a man—whatever his problems.

In the novel *Dr. Giovanni*, Arturo Vivanti describes his quest for the woman with whom he can—finally—lose his virginity. He meets a beautiful woman to whom he is attracted and indebted because she is also a muse.

> "Age doesn't matter," she had said. But to me it did matter. The phrase, I thought, had value only when the younger of the two said it, and I pondered over and counted her years, and now she was twenty, not sixty and more. . . . I brought an arm over my eyes and frowned while her velvety, clever hand glided and swept over mine like a moth. I must go, I thought. I tried to get up. But desire kept me pinned to the bed. In the dark, I thought, didn't she look as though she were twenty? Didn't she look just like the portrait of her as a girl, that I could see dimly there on the tripod? And who was more desirable than she? It was true, she was—must be—over sixty, but she was extraordinary. . . .[18]

She was not extraordinary *enough* to be worthy of this young man. He lived in a culture where the remark, "Age does not matter," is naturally interpreted by a man to mean that she has taken upon herself the power to nullify the social evaluation of her passage out of the state of fertility. It does not occur to him for one minute that she is telling him that *his* age, his inexperience, is not important. She is simply too old to represent the feminine ideal with which he must couple.

In our culture a woman is sexually desirable only as long as her sexuality can also inspire fear. Once she no longer menstruates she is assumed to have lost her sexuality. This assumption is projection, of course. She has not lost *her* sexuality, but man has lost a great deal of his sexual interest in her—a distinction which is not commonly understood.

Men consider menstruating women sexy and menopausal woman sexless. Like other male myths about female sexuality, this will go unchallenged as long as women remain ignorant about the actual facts of life. For example, an older woman who finds that her mate is no longer taking sexual initiative may see this decline as proof that she has, indeed, lost her sexuality. But, in fact, this may mean that he is less able to act on his sexual interest than he was when *he* was younger:

> In advising her how to relieve local discomfort during intercourse, the physician must not overlook such psychological components as those related to the diminished libido and reduced potency of the husband. The uninformed wife may believe herself rejected or be alarmed by the increasing physical effort to achieve sexual satisfaction unless she is reassuringly apprised of the customary loss of male sexual vigor. She should be told of her husband's probable desperation concerning his problem.[19]

If her mate is honest, the menopausal woman will not be blamed for his loss of sexual ability. More often than not, however, she is blamed, consciously or unconsciously, and our culture gives the opportunity to observe the common sort of "courage" shown by men during this change in their lives. He is likely to reject his partner (at least temporarily) and seek a "golden" girl who will restore his youthful virility.

The common rationalization of such actions is that women are no longer interested in sex after menopause. This rationalization, of course, is presented in the form of a "truth" and many women have themselves come to believe it.

What does a woman go through? Everything I've ever heard about seems to imply that after a woman has been through the menopause, her sex life isn't satisfying. She turns frigid. (K.B., *age sixteen*)

As long as a woman remains healthy and her body is not deprived of sufficient estrogen, she remains sexually healthy, as capable of enjoying her sexual life as she was before menopause. Indeed, Clara Thompson points out that:

> Many women have a kind of rebirth after menopause. Their general health is better. Freed from concern about possible pregnancy, their

sex lives often become more spontaneous and satisfying. Although there is no longer the fiery passion of youth, sex becomes expressive of a tried and trusted companionship and intimacy often more satisfactory in its total meaning than earlier experiences.[20]

Theoretically, at least, women are able to enjoy a more rewarding sex life after menopause. No doubt many women are enjoying the fruits of their age even while acting as if sex were the last thing that interests them. Many other women may indeed lose interest in sex simply because they believe that it is what ought to be happening to them at "that time of life." And then there are women who know they are capable of enjoying sex and who are ready to enjoy the intimacy of which Thompson speaks, only to find that their mates of years standing need to find a younger woman.

Our society easily accepts this kind of solution as long as it is employed by men. The coupling of the older man with a younger woman is absolutely acceptable. However, should an older woman begin a sexual relationship with a younger man, she is seen as a new sort of libertine, and everyone wonders what the young man is "getting" out of it. In purely sexual terms, of course, the young man is likely to find in his older partner a woman who has realized her capacity for sexual response, while the young woman is likely to find in her older partner a man who has a diminished capacity for sexual response. But biological fact, as we have already seen, is often twisted or obliterated to serve social ends. This particular biological fact is totally ignored while society continues to believe that older women are not sexual, and the coupling of an older woman and younger man is perverse.

To many of us, a woman who seems sexual after menopause is a deviant. She is still expected to fulfill the male image of woman which, after menopause, means her sexuality has disappeared. In our culture most women submit to this definition of femininity and pretend to have no sexuality, thereby giving support to the male projection. Vivian Gornick, in her book *In Search of Ali Mahmoud*, reports on a different perspective:

> What was great in the midst of all this madness was the sexiness of the women, the older women acting as sexy and drunkenly self-assured as the younger women. Women of fifty behaving as though they considered themselves as desirable as their twenty-five-year-old daughters. And, indeed, they were, the men caressing and courting them as often as they did the younger women; and the older women responding or

ignoring, accepting or repelling, with the same degree of lustful vanity that their daughters displayed. If I had gone up to one of these be-wigged Melina Mercouris and said to her, "Listen, where I come from they put you in a closet when you pass thirty-five and any woman who then acts as you're doing now does so out of nervous desperation, and everyone feels contempt and pity, like she doesn't know her *place*," she would surely have looked as though I were mildly retarded, and if she could have she would have replied, "But I do not understand. I am alive, no? And while I desire I am desirable, no?"

I never again in Egypt saw women quite like that, but I never forgot those women, either. To this day, when I recall that party I feel pleasure, and somewhere inside myself I am crowing. Because there it was in all its blowsy, full-blown possibility.[21]

What if a woman in our culture is an iconoclast and refuses to "act her age," to pretend she is not sexual? And what happens if she also refuses to bow to convention and has a sexual relationship with a young man? A partial answer to these questions is suggested in Hal Ashby's movie *Harold and Maude*. Maude (age seventy-nine) and Harold (about twenty) fall in love, have a sexual relationship, and Harold declares his wish to marry her.

Mother, of course, thinks it's a bizarre notion; a sentiment echoed and enhanced by the representatives of the social order: the army officer (visually supported by a photograph of the President), the psychoanalyst (flanked by a picture of Freud), and the priest (supported by the framed image of the Pope). The priest tells Harold that he is revolted by the image of this young man's "firm young body commingling with the withered flesh, the sagging breasts," and so on, of this woman, and he concludes the sermon by saying, it "makes me want to vomit."

One is forced to compare these responses with the images in any number of movies where Maurice Chevalier, for example, doted on the firm-fleshed countenance of a young woman. No comments were made about the discrepancies of physiognomy or attitude—none were considered "necessary." Attitudes toward the sexuality of older women have not changed since the time her image was articulated by Eckharth.

Maude, an extraordinary woman, gets her man and enjoys her sexuality into her seventy-ninth year. We do not know the ways in which societal reactions would have dimmed her pleasure. (She kills herself on her eightieth birthday as she had planned many years before.) Perhaps she would have been oblivious to these pressures, since she had ignored so many conventions earlier. But, while she is a delightful character, Maude is not one with whom easy identification is possible—her self-confidence is limitless and ironclad.

Most women become sexually invisible after menopause, not because of any mysterious or well-known physical upheaval but because the culture expects them to. The competition for a mate, the high value placed upon being young (i.e., attractive) is so great that many young women would, indeed, respond to a sexy postmenopausal woman with pity for her desperate hour.* If the young woman is going to "get the goodies" she has been promised in exchange for giving up autonomy, she is going to want as little competition as possible. This becomes another reason why women are reluctant to extend their notion of sisterhood past the age of menopause. The results, of course, include the reinforcement of the idea that woman's life ends with menopause; and so the younger woman herself becomes desperate to reap her rewards while she still can. She believes in the myth of menopause, and she capitalizes on it until age takes away her ability to do so.

In most situations the menopausal woman, aware of the ways in which she is perceived, feels forced to hide or disguise her sexuality. She pretends that sex no longer interests her. If she hopes to "keep" her mate, she is expected to devote herself to the task of regenerating his potency. She is naturally spurred to perform these emotional contortions by the environment which has made the probability of her finding a more suitable mate small and the reprisals for seeking one large. Sometimes, however, even the implied threats (whether of ostracism or loneliness) are not enough—the pretense hardly seems worthwhile.

Part of the menopausal disguise is the denial of sexuality; the remainder consists of continuing to act as though the feelings and needs of a man (and/or children) are more important than her own. In the character of Maude we saw a woman whose needs meshed with those of Harold—one was not made happy at the expense of the other. But again, Maude was an extraordinary woman, she spent her life being herself as she defined it, and Harold wasn't exactly a commonplace type either.

Most women come to menopause with a lifetime of pretense behind them and little idea of their own needs. They have lived with

*It is no surprise in this connection that the audience with which I saw *Harold and Maude* laughed at Maude the first time she gave Harold a seductive look.

the desire to make a man happy and to consider the needs of husband and children before their own. Such a woman is well portrayed by Doris Lessing in *The Summer Before the Dark*. Shortly after the novel begins, Kate Brown, a "well-preserved" upper-class English-woman, experiences a profound change in her being. As Lessing describes it, "the light that was the desire to please had gone out." This light, which women are taught to tend from puberty, is the source of energy for the many manipulations women must perform to remain feminine—that is, sexually desirable—objects. The light went out for Kate Brown, but not as a result of her own choice.

> The small chill wind was blowing very definitely, if still softly enough; this was the first time in her life that she was not wanted. She was unnecessary. That this time in her life was approaching she had of course known very well for years. She had even made plans for it; she would study this, travel there, take up this or that type of welfare work. It is not possible, after all, to be a woman with any sort of mind, and not know that in middle age, in the full flood of one's capacities and energies, one is bound to become that well-documented and much studied phenomenon, the woman with grown-up children and not enough to do, whose energies must be switched from the said children to less vulnerable targets, for everybody's sake, for her own as well as theirs. So there was nothing surprising about what was happening. Perhaps she ought to have expected it sooner?
>
> She had not expected it this summer. Next summer, or the year after that, yes, but not now. What she had set herself to face had been all in the future.[22]

Kate Brown, caught by surprise, is abandoned. Her husband and children go off on summer-long trips, and there is no need for her to maintain a fully operating household. Kate "lets herself go" as she was let go. No longer looking like an attractive (sexual) woman of forty-odd years, and fearing after a time that perhaps she has strayed too far, Kate Brown decides to give the world of male approval another try.

> . . . She hurried herself into one of summer's beautiful dresses, bones inside a tent, tried to push her hair closer to her head, and gave up, then went out into the street. Under the street lamps, groups of young men hung about, hoping that something would happen; the pubs must have just closed.
>
> She thought, *I can't, I can't* go past them; for each group of men, even a couple of young boys standing by themselves, seemed threaten-ing. But she forced herself, a self-prescribed corrective to a need to

dive back down into the flat, pull blankets over her head, and stay there. The street seemed wide, endless, each object in its embodied danger; she seemed to herself all vulnerable surfaces. She walked, with her eyes straight ahead, as she would in Italy or Spain, where women are made to feel overexposed, roped off like municipal grass; *Keep Off.*

No one took any notice. She received indifferent glances, which turned off her at once, in search of stimulus.

Again, she might have been invisible.

Her whole surface, the shields of her blank, staring eyes, her body, even her trimly set feet, had been set to receive notice, like an adolescent girl who has spent three hours making up and who staked everything on what will happen when she presents herself to batteries of searchlight eyes. Kate felt light, floating, without ballast; her head was chaotic, her feelings numb with confusion, she was suppressing impulses so far from anything she had ever had, or could have imagined as hers, that she was shocked by them as if reading about them in a newspaper: she knew that if she were not careful she would march up to one of those groups of lolling men and lift her skirts or expose herself: "*There*, look at that, I'm here, can't you see? Why don't you look at me?"[23]

Women quite rightly want to take control of the conditions in which they will be sexual. The fact remains that it will not be easy to give up the small advantages we now have—even the ones that currently seem like liabilities. We want to be less visible on the street. But if, like Kate Brown, we arrive at a state in which we are invisible, the experience is shockingly unpleasant.

What could more easily drive a woman to the point of breakdown than to find herself at an arbitrary, biologically defined point in her life stripped of her identity as a sexual being? No wonder that Kate's response was to want to lift her skirts and assert that she was indeed a woman.

We have seen (in chapters 4 and 7) that psychoanalysts have paid little theoretical attention to menopausal woman, either in terms of her own psychology or that of men in relation to menopause. Their lack of theory has not, however, kept some analysts from expounding on the status of women once menstruation stops. Helene Deutsch says:

At the moment when expulsion of ova from the ovary ceases, all organic processes devoted to the service of the species stop. Woman has ended her existence as bearer of a new future, and has reached her natural end—her partial death—as servant of the species. She is now engaged in an active struggle against her decline.

Woman's biologic fate manifests itself in the disappearance of her individual feminine qualities at the same time that her service to the species ceases. As we have said, everything she acquired during puberty is now lost piece by piece: with the lapse of the reproductive service, her beauty vanishes, and usually the warm, vital flow of her feminine emotional life as well.[24]

Deutsch sees herself as a student of the human condition, not a cultural commentator. She tells this story of menopause as though it were obviously true that women's emotional (sexual) life naturally ends when they no longer ovulate. Her vision, interestingly enough, is quite similar to that of Simone de Beauvoir, whose starting point in observation is quite different: ". . . When the first hints come of that fated and irreversible process which is to destroy the whole edifice built up during puberty, she feels the fatal touch of death itself."[25] Deutsch talks about the "acquisitions" of puberty, which are assumed to have been blessings, while de Beauvoir calls the same process the building up of an edifice. Each continues her analysis of the possibilities open to a woman at the time of menopause:

> Successful psychotherapy in the climacterium is made difficult be-
> cause usually there is little one can offer to the patient as a substitute
> for the fantasy gratifications. There is a large element of real fear
> behind the neurotic anxiety, for reality has actually become poor in
> prospects, and resignation without compensation is often the only
> solution. And resignation is the hardest task for a human being![26]

And de Beauvoir:

> Here we come upon the sorry tragedy of the aged woman; she realizes
> she is useless, all her life long the middle class woman has often had
> to solve the ridiculous problem of how to kill time. But when the
> children are grown, the husband a made man or at least settled down,
> the time must still be killed somehow. Fancy work was invented to
> mask their horrible idleness; hands embroider, they knit, they are in
> motion. This is no real work, for the object reproduced is trifling, and
> to know what to do with it is often a problem. . . . This is no longer
> a game that in its uselessness expressed the pure joy of living; and it is
> hardly an escape, since the mind remained vacant. It is the "absurd
> amusement" described by Pascal; with the needle of the crochet hook,
> woman sadly weaves the very nothingness of her days.[27]

Deutsch, the psychoanalyst, tells us that her discipline is not of very much use to menopausal women. Where "nature" has cut off the possibility of further development, analysis can offer no further guidance. This is a sad example of the ways in which psychoanalysis performs the most conservative function because its earliest writers confused biology with destiny and psyche with culture. The purpose of de Beauvoir's bitter examination was to make clear to women that the society must be changed, rather than to suggest that women must "adjust" themselves to the loss of an effective life upon the decay of the ovaries.

It is possible for women to begin a second career, as it were, after menopause. It is happening right now. However, if women continue to accept the common social definition of femininity and its demise at menopause, the careers begun after menopause will be only one small step removed from the busywork de Beauvoir has described. Such second careers will more often than not be compensatory rather than a new source of fulfillment. One can still do "something," but something is a world removed from substance.

In some cases, the social world accepts skilled or semiskilled labor as fit and proper work only for a man. In this context, the work for which a woman is prepared (which most probably will require no skills) will be seen as substantial, and the job market open.*

The woman who approaches menopause while living in an environment where only professionals are respected finds herself in an almost impossible situation. The training required for such work takes years of expensive schooling. She may find that volunteer work is the only thing available that meets any of her demands but, because there is no money attached to it, her efforts may not seem real.

If women choose to be full-time mothers, they must understand that at most this can only be considered a first career. (The women who were taught that motherhood is a lifetime job, after all, contribute to the statistics on middle-aged depression.) Motherhood is not generally considered a relevant experience for women who enter the job market. It is important to understand and deal with this before one's second career is imminent.

Many women have learned this under great stress and with few options. There are other women who have come to menopause with a long period of serious involvement in nondomestic work behind them, although some have found that the menopausal woman is no more desirable in many job situations than she is as a "sex object."

---

* This will be particularly true as long as women are given less pay for the same work as a man. Such women represent a large new source of cheap labor.

When the taboo lifts at menopause, a woman is given the freedom to become a self-defined person (a freedom denied young women), but all too often this takes on the same quality as being all dressed up with no place to go. The self-confidence gained after menopause meets with the bitter reality that no one is terribly responsive to its existence. It has, perhaps, come too late.

As a young woman grows she ought to learn that the menstrual phase of her life, the fertile years, is in fact only one phase of her development, neither the acme of biological identity nor the only time of life that has meaning. It is cruel and unreasonable not to educate young women to believe that twenty-five or more years of life exist beyond the time of fertility and cyclicity.

Older women can contribute to the education of the young, but to do this (and thereby effectively increase female opportunities) they must reveal more than we have heretofore seen. For the most part, mothers, sisters, friends, teachers have all been silent. Famous women have also been silent.

Younger women can marvel at the accomplishments of Margaret Mead, Simone de Beauvoir,* or Antonia Brico,† and perhaps use these women as models. But one cannot easily identify with them, since they are portrayed or portray themselves as exceptional and extraordinary. We haven't a clue to the ways in which these particular women or most older women feel during the transition from fertility to post-menopause. Because of this, the younger woman is free to believe the myths that haunt her and provoke her to wish menopause would never come. One may assume, because these women are still vital and hardworking, that nothing too dreadful befell them during this transition, but we cannot be *sure.*

It is perhaps a male idea that accomplishment is enough, that we need only to admire, or envy, or dream of equaling a person who is successful. It is, perhaps, a female idea that we need to know more—that we want to know the everyday details of someone's life as well as those details which make it extraordinary.

So imbued am I with this "male" idea that I feel it presumptuous or ridiculous to ask that women of note talk about menopause and ageing and tell us how they have felt. And who can be sure that very

---

* De Beauvoir has written about ageing but not about her menopause.
† *Antonia: Portrait of the Woman,* a movie made by Judy Collins and Jill Godmilow, shows a generous spirit as well as an accomplished conductor at work in her seventy-third year.

much would be gained by the exposure of "private" and personal experience? The only thing we can be sure of is what has been lost through ignorance.

Girl children will have everything to gain when they grow up in a society in which the menstrual taboo is discussed. When women are no longer affected by the taboo—and for this to happen, they must talk openly to one another—the great differences we now perceive before and after menopause will disappear. If menopause is to become an integrated part of life rather than the separate crisis it now is, women must define and share their own experiences.

10

Changes

One who has lived many years in a city, as soon as she goes to sleep,
Beholds another city full of good and evil, and her own city vanishes
*   from her mind.*
She does not say to herself, "This is a new city: I am a stranger here";
Nay, she thinks she has always lived in this city and was born and bred
*   in it.*
What wonder, then, if the soul does not remember her ancient abode
*   and birthplace,*
Since she is wrapt in the slumber of this world, like a star covered by
*   clouds?—*
Especially as she has trodden so many cities and the dust that darkens
*   her vision is not yet swept away.*
                                    —JALAL-UD-DIN RUMI (1207–1273)

Menstruation and menopause are a dirty deal; the taboo has
caused women to believe that there is no special value, no advantage
or superiority to be gained from the process of cyclicity, or any
benefit to be derived from the discreet changes that mark the transition from puberty to cyclicity and from cyclicity to post-menopause.
It has led us to believe that we would, in fact, be better off without a
hormone system that differs from men's, as though the functioning
of male sex hormones were the superior model from which to make
judgments.

It is a precept of feminism that women control their own bodies
and have a maximum opportunity for choice. Sixty-nine percent of
the women who responded to the menstrual questionnaire said that
given the choice they would rather not menstruate. While the remaining 31 percent enjoy menstruation and feel it to be a confirmation of healthy functioning or of femininity, the fact remains that
more than two out of every three women (and presumably people
with an active interest in women's liberation)* would do away with
menstruation provided that it could be done safely and they could
still remain fertile. If menstruation were completely suppressed, the
level of female sex hormones would be altered in such a way that the
transition from fertile to post-fertile levels would probably no longer

* This is based on the fact that respondents to the questionnaire were readers of
  Ms. magazine or friends of readers.

be the occasion for a major change in hormone production. Menopause would become a minor biochemical event.

The desire to be free of menstruation and, presumably, menopause, might be interpreted as a progressive step toward liberation—an instance in which women are exercising control over their own bodies. In my opinion, however, this preference is not really an indication of an informed free choice but results from the pressures exerted by the menstrual taboo.

Thousands of years of history and the history of their own experience have led women to their present opinion that menstruation and menopause are fundamentally unacceptable parts of life and must be ignored as important biological events. Compared with primitive practices, the modern-day version of the taboo makes social and emotional change particularly difficult.

In many primitive cultures the taboo presented women with grave difficulties. Among the Lele of the Congo, for example:

> . . . a menstruating woman was a danger to the whole community if she entered the forest. Not only was her menstruation certain to wreck any enterprise in the forest that she might undertake, but it was thought to produce unfavorable conditions for men. Hunting would be difficult for a long time after, and rituals based on forest plants would have no efficacy. Women found these rules extremely irksome, especially as they were regularly short-handed and late in their planting, weeding, harvesting and fishing.[1]

The Lele women were annoyed—an understandable response to the rules which clearly limited their actions. Had they dared to overturn the taboo, however, they would have had concrete evidence to prove that it existed and hampered their way of life. Although the practice of the taboo was probably not uniformly oppressive to women, it was uniformly evident.

While those women who were isolated in menstrual huts were similarly constrained and perhaps similarly annoyed, they were temporarily freed from daily chores and responsibilities, free to share each other's company, perhaps to sing together, tell stories, and make objects of craft. They also had the benefit of *knowing* that their community believed they were unclean.

In our culture, where the rules of taboo are not articulated and there is little information about the positive experiences of menstruation and menopause, confusion and difficulty are bound to prevail. Instead of protesting the contemporary version of the taboo, women, unaware of its existence, protest the "problem" of menstruation and its legacy, menopause. Instead of protesting against the societal attitudes that created the taboo, we are attacking our own bodies and that portion of female identity which presents us with the "problem."

In most cases it appears that the desire to be free from menstruation, the menstrual cycle, and menopause arises from the belief that these processes are a biological impediment. The responses to two questions in the menstrual survey reveal the feelings of those women who "choose" to be rid of cyclicity, blood, and menopause. When asked "Do women have an advantage because they menstruate?" and "Do men have any advantage because they do not menstruate?" 71 percent said menstruation brings women no advantage and 63 percent that men are advantaged because they do not menstruate.

Of the women who believed that men were at an advantage because they don't menstruate, only 10 percent gave as their reason the freedom from the social stigma associated with menstruation. The majority of women said that the major advantage was in the "freedom from inconvenience or mess," "freedom from cramps," or said men didn't have to spend the "extra time or money." Most of the women considered menstruation a biological liability and believed that men are in a superior position because they have a more advantageous (i.e., superior) biological makeup!

In stating these opinions women are giving evidence of a tacit acceptance of the menstrual taboo and its misconceptions. They are saying that menstruation and menopause are biological infirmities and are marks of sexual disadvantage (inferiority)—menstruation is a drag and menopause a disaster. ("Drag" and "disaster" being the equivalents, in this case, of the more old-fashioned word "unclean.")

The powers of sisterhood have not yet been strong enough to overthrow the prejudices of the taboo. Large numbers of women who consider themselves proponents of women's liberation are accepting a male definition of a fundamental female experience. Women might do well to review the experience of other contemporary groups who have sought liberation and who have carefully examined the ways in which prejudice directed toward their members takes place. One aspect of this analysis is the study of the relationship between power and identity. Powerlessness and a weak sense of identity go hand in hand. That Black and Red are now beautiful is the result of a reaffirmed self-respect that had been decimated by oppression.

In general, women have only taken a partial look into the relationship between power and identity. Thus far, we have concentrated on those arenas from which we were unjustly excluded and have worked to rectify the resulting inequities. But we have shied away from a more careful analysis of femininity. In so doing, women have responded quite uniquely to the threat of co-optation represented by the liberal community and the threat of backlash from the old-fashioned sexist.

It has been customary for liberals to respond to movements for liberation with the statement that these are laudable endeavors but "only" special cases of the general quest for human rights—a quest in which we are all "equally" interested. To propose that we all have an equal stake and interest in the formation of an egalitarian global village is at best a fancy of privilege which the powerless might find laughable or enraging. It is curious to note, however, that in the sphere of sexual injustice, both the powerful and the powerless are in agreement—at least where the deeper issues of femininity in general are concerned and menstruation and menopause in particular. It appears that both sexes believe menstruation and menopause are nuisances at the very least, and both believe that women would be "better" or more equal if they didn't have "peculiar" (female) sex hormones. Women have precipitously agreed with the liberal position that we are all alike—or at least *ought* to be. We have prematurely tried to smooth out the rocky road to equality and have come to believe that if our hormones are different, they "don't really count," or, if they insist on making themselves (and ourselves) obvious, they ought to be done away with.

While it may reassure the powerful that being human is synonymous with being alike and that we all want and need the same things, this is, in the end, untrue. If the global village is not diverse, it will be peopled with individuals whose homogeneity is defined and determined by those who have the power to bring it into existence.

It is more problematic and cumbersome to move toward liberation while remaining aware of sexual differences, especially if these qualities and values are not respected by those in power, but the potential gains are great. The menstrual taboo prevents women from experiencing the full dimension of being female. It is the essence of the experience that makes the struggle for freedom truly worth our while—not only for ourselves as individuals but for the world in which the next generations will live.

> It would be a thousand pities if women wrote like men, or lived like men, or looked like men, for if two sexes are quite inadequate, considering the vastness and variety of the world, how should we manage with one only? Ought not education to bring out and fortify the dif-

ferences rather than the similarities? For we have too much likeness as it is, and if an explorer should come and bring work of other sexes looking through the branches of other trees at other skies, nothing would be of greater service to humanity; and we should have the immense pleasure in the bargain of watching professor "X" rush for his measuring-rods to prove himself "superior."[2]

While Virginia Woolf's detached humor here is enticing, it is often beyond us, living as we do in a world seemingly filled with Professor "X's." As soon as a sexual difference is noted, it generally follows that those in a more advantaged position need to judge it and find that *their* difference is in fact the superior one. This form of backlash is one we quite naturally fear; after all, what is the point of women defining sexual difference if men are only to say that each difference is the mark of female inferiority?

The desire to sidestep the issue of sexual difference is understandable, but it is quite literally self-defeating. As Margaret Mead says:

Our tendency at present is to minimize all these differences that are seen as handicaps on one sex. . . . But every adjustment that minimizes a difference, a vulnerability, in one sex, a differential strength in the other, diminishes their possibility of complementing each other. . . .

Guard each sex in its vulnerable moments we must, protect and cherish them through the crises that at some times are so much harder for one sex than for the other. But as we guard, we may also keep the differences. Simply compensating for differences is in the end a form of denial. . . .[3]

The male definition of femininity created a prison, but woman's denial of any sexual difference that influences personality and the compensations issuing thence creates the walls of a new prison. It may look more modern and its facilities may be greatly improved, but it is still a jail.

With respect to menstruation and menopause, the penal institution is formed by the menstrual taboo, and the walls are made from shame of feelings of inferiority. Bravado or denial change the appearance but not the substance of this jail, which is women's low opinion of femininity and sexual identity.

In order to change the social evaluation of women it is necessary to change our attitudes about the biological and emotional foundations of female existence, as well as our attitudes toward cyclicity and modes of hormone variation. It is impossible to do this completely and thoroughly while living as members of a society that will not accept the existence of women as different and equal. So it will therefore be necessary to take a long-range view, working toward change while accepting the inevitability that this will be partial but can continue to evolve in future generations. However, one might choose to accelerate the evolutionary process of change by removing oneself as completely as possible from the stream of the society which needs alteration. It is the latter view that serves as rationale and possible motive for the various separatist movements.

In the women's movement, radical feminists and/or radical lesbian feminists have told us that Men (if not men as individuals) are the enemy of progress in the struggle for women's full emancipation, and that to achieve liberation we must remove ourselves from the world of men (and perhaps from intimate contact with men as well). The construction of the menstrual taboo and its maintenance are in part products of the man's world and the male need to project onto women that which is uncomfortable to live with in the male self. It is therefore impossible to argue with the view that change will come only in rejecting these values.

Separatism in its more severe form, that of sexuality and intimacy, is less simple to agree with. While sexual attraction may be altered or modified by political belief or personal needs, it is extremely unlikely that the gender of one's partner will be determined by one's politics. Indeed, in connection with attitudes toward menstruation and menopause even celibacy would not provide a solution since both men and women share the legacy of the menstrual taboo. At the outset at least, both partners are likely to feel that menstruation is a drag and menopause a disaster.

Separatism, however, has enabled some women to confront the issues of femininity in a less reactive manner. For example, it has given some lesbian women the desire to observe and understand menstruation and menopause in a new light. I received a long letter from a traveling lesbian commune in which the women recounted the individual experiences and menstrual histories of the members and described the pattern of menstrual synchrony that had evolved as they lived and traveled together. Recently I went to a concert where I heard a song about menstruation which celebrated the monthly flow of blood and suggested that by sharing our experience we will remove the curse and leave the pleasures. It closed with the message that lesbianism is the "solution" to the problem of male denigration of menstruating woman.

It is presumptuous to consider lesbianism as a solution for anything other than a woman's desire for exclusive sexual relations with other women. The excesses of women who seek to promote lesbianism as a political rather than a sexual choice ought not blind us to the value of the insights lesbian feminists are sharing. These women are often the first to reconsider freely the highly charged matter of being female. Furthermore, they can help heterosexual women to understand the extent to which fear of men's opinion and male power limits the search for self-knowledge.

The menstrual taboo has influenced every thought and every feeling about menstruation, menopause, and being a woman. The taboo is virulent, its presence felt by all of us, although we cannot point to an edifice in which it is contained. We cannot know all the changes that will take place in our lives when the taboo no longer exists, but we can assume that by naming it for what it is, change will begin. From this starting place we can go on to speculate, to imagine life without the taboo, and we can begin to give this new life its shape.

The women's movement as a collective force has not yet focused on the issues of menstruation and menopause or on the physiological and emotional repercussions of these cycles. However, there are women whose interest in feminism has led to the establishment of forums in which these issues can be investigated, and some investigation has already begun.

Consciousness-raising groups have allowed women to examine many heretofore assumed "realities" of female life, and the illusions on which they have rested have been exposed. The model of consciousness-raising has been used for women's groups formed around specific issues, including those of menstruation and menopause. A menopause group, for example, was formed by a small group of women in California. After meeting regularly once a week, one of the women came in and reported a "strange" experience. The hot flushes she had been experiencing had occurred once again, but this time she found them pleasurable!

I doubt that many women anticipate or experience pleasurable hot flushes; but then not many of us have talked about them, thought about them, or questioned our assumptions about them. And not many of us have had the experience of being members of a group that supports a new view of a very old subject.

In some groups, women keep menstrual calendars, and other women outside the group are encouraged to do the same. People may begin to keep records for their daughters or friends and then show them the results. I have kept track of the cycles of my closest friends who claimed they never experienced any cyclic changes. After a couple of months, I handed them the evidence and they finally realized that some of their feelings were indeed predictable and patterned.

If many groups of women kept menstrual records and continued to note how they felt during the menopause, in ten or twenty years we would have longitudinal records for thousands and thousands of women. Once pooled, analyzed, and then publicized, all of us would finally have a solid idea of the range of normal experience, how it varies between individuals. In this way, we would have our own guide to our own experience.

Once women give the subjects of menstruation and menopause greater credence, a forum will exist in which the issues associated with these cycles can be challenged and examined. This is as true for overriding general issues as it is for highly specific ones. For example, one of the women who responded to the questionnaire sent along a fact sheet provided by a hostel association. They, in turn, had used information provided by the Parks Department in making the following warning: "Special precautions apply to women. For their protection, women should refrain from wilderness travel during their menstrual periods. Bears and other large carnivores have attacked women in this physiological condition." For thousands (perhaps millions) of women, the parks service warning if obeyed means a curtailment of recreational activity. For women whose work takes them to wilderness areas, this warning represents economic and professional hardship. This admonition to stay out of the forest is reminiscent of the Lele taboo, although in this instance, at least, the danger is said to exist for women and not all of society. To do away with the taboo it is imperative that the matter does not rest here; pressure must be applied for further research.

Another specific issue that a group formed around the topic of menstruation or menopause might begin to explore is that of ageing: how women are affected by society's views, and how women of different ages affect one another. The general view is that menstruation has a diffuse influence on a woman's life (albeit a negative one). It is her curse, but one so pervasive that it would not be worthwhile to study it. There is no attention given to menstruation that is not a sidelong glance at an unpleasant aspect of femininity. Menopause, however, is seen as a discrete event; it is a medical and social problem. Menopause is a crisis, menstruation an ongoing aspect of female life.

The result of these attitudes is that women tend to believe that there is no need to pay attention to menstruation (except when there is a huge problem), while a great deal of attention and tension should be directed toward menopause. Within the women's movement, for example, there has been little analysis of the cycles of life and the ways in which one stage of life leads to the next. We have been guilty of age discrimination by not studying the continuities and commonalities but focusing instead on the crises.

Small women's groups are often the precursors of women's centers. In larger numbers, women can join with those who have the same special interests and concentrate on one area. Many women have now taken courses such as Know Your Body or Our Bodies, Our Selves, and then go on to teach courses of their own. Sometimes still more specialized groups then emerge naturally out of the experience of sharing knowledge and information. The experience of the women in the Boston Women's Health Collective, for example, led to the book Our Bodies, Our Selves, which has helped thousands of women.* The Women's Health Organizing Collective in New York City wrote a series of pamphlets, one most memorably entitled How to Get Through the Maze with Your Feet in the Stirrups (a consumer guide to gynecology clinics in lower Manhattan).

Other projects have begun. Women in many communities have started to monitor private as well as public gynecological services. Ratings of gynecologists are available to women throughout the community. Really terrible doctors can be boycotted, but even more effective is the technique of confronting the doctor with his rating. (A boycott runs the risk of steering informed women from the doctor, while others will find that he has lots of office time to give them.)

If a group confronts a gynecologist or hospital administrator with the reports of other women, he or she is likely to be moved—just a little. Doctors need patients, after all, and administrators don't want to lose tax funds.

Through techniques like these, hospitals and private physicians can be encouraged to offer more comprehensive medical care to women and to treat the problems of menstruation and menopause, as well as the healthy functioning of these processes, with greater respect.

At a recent meeting of a newly formed women's center, the question of installing a toilet was under discussion. A friend turned to me and said that as soon as the bathroom was working, we'd have to make sure that tampons and napkins were for sale.

* A revised edition, containing responses to a menopause questionnaire, will be published during the winter of 1975/76.

Wait a minute, I thought. *For Sale?* Why should we consider them a luxury item, for heaven's sake; we wouldn't think of charging anyone for toilet paper or soap. The government treats menstrual paraphernalia as a luxury and taxes it, but we should not make the same mistake or accept theirs any longer. Why should any public toilet facility or any place of business that has toilets charge for tampons and napkins? Women have been speaking out against the nonsense of pay toilets; we might well include the ridiculousness of people acting as though menstrual needs were an "extra."

I wrote to the companies that manufacture all these products, asking for information. I didn't receive the kind of information I wanted (what percentage of women use pads, for example). Several weeks after my letters went out, packages began to arrive. I brought them home, wondering what was inside, and opened them to find colorful cardboard boxes. In turn these were opened and inside each box was an assortment of the full line of menstrually related products manufactured by a given company—pads, tampons, belts, panties.

I was surprised by these packages but even more surprised by my reaction. Instead of appraising them purely as public relations offerings, for the first time ever I felt that menstruation was *special*. I don't doubt that my response to "gifts" might be called sentimental, but it was an important feeling for me. Only when something special and good came to me solely because I menstruate did I realize that menstruation could be a pleasurable aspect of life. Attention was paid to it, not because of its discomforts but simply because it happens.

It is not surprising that the people who profit from menstruation have found it worthwhile to experiment with new ways of treating the subject. There is no doubt that changes in the paraphernalia associated with menstruation have contributed toward and reinforced changes in women's attitude toward flow and the female body. Forty or fifty years ago, women used rags to catch menstrual blood. Each day of bleeding the rags were washed, hung up to dry, and fresh ones had to be made.

My grandmother told me that her mother told her that if a man saw a woman's menstrual flow he would go blind. (I thought that was hilarious.) She also told me that when she started to menstruate, no one had told her anything about menstruation and she was very frightened. She said that women used clean rags to blot the flow. I felt myself very lucky to have sanitary napkins. (A.K.)

Ten or fifteen years ago, most of us used sanitary napkins. They were an improvement on rags, but.

When I was fifteen and a half (fifteen years ago), we traveled by car on a trip. When we stopped at a motel my father removed the suitcase that contained our overnight things. I had a box of Kotex in a paper sack and asked him to take that in, too. He said, "What is it?" I said, "Just take it in." I was embarrassed that he was handling it and angry that he was also embarrassed and questioned me. He was red in the face and handled the sack as though it was dirty pictures or something. Neither of us at that point regarded menstruation or its paraphernalia as normal, everyday occurrences.   (M.E.)

We girls, barred from swimming, banished from touch football, constantly adjusting our belts and pads, consistently being caught without the proper paraphernalia in the middle of a school day, constantly losing safety pins down the john, soon learned to call it the "curse."

(J.C.B.)

The "sexual revolution" brought a changing emphasis on virginity. Although tampons can be used and the hymen remain intact, tampons were considered a threat to virginity until virginity was no longer an essential precursor to a happily married life. Women who are now out of their teens and not yet past menopause came to menarche during the time of transition in which virginity was losing, but had not quite lost, its cosmic character. We started out with pads, and then, years later, many switched to tampons.

I wish my mother had known more about Tampax. She only knew about napkins and I spent the first twelve years of my period with napkins—she thought Tampax was only for "married women" (non-virgins), yet she used them only two years before menopause. My attitude toward menstruation has changed dramatically since using internal tampons. I feel very good about touching myself, putting in my diaphragm and dealing with my period since I learned about tampons. Menstruating is really no chore—it's rather exciting to be a woman!   (J.M.L.)

I do not feel that menstruation is a bother since I started to use tampons. I feel as though they have changed my ideas toward menstruation. Pads and belts were so hectic, uncomfortable and unbearable!

(D.S.)

One of the most liberating days of my life was the day I was able to

insert a tampon. It took many tries and many tears. I just didn't know
where it should go. I was sixteen!   (K.F.T.)

In the past ten years there has been a proliferation of products.
Now there are many brands, each providing a range of napkins and
tampons and each with a feature that is touted as a major breakthrough in the sphere of "feminine hygiene." The number of variations on the market gives us a greater choice than we had, but they
are not providing the dramatic change many of us experienced when
we went from pads to tampons. Only one new product has been
developed in recent years—a flexible cup that is put into the vagina to
collect the blood. Depending on the volume of flow, it can stay in
place for a few hours or the entire day. When full, it is discarded and
a new cup inserted.

When I switched from Kotex to tampons, I couldn't imagine why
anyone continued to use sanitary napkins. Now that I'm using the
infinitely more convenient and cleaner Tassaway cups, I can't imagine
why anyone continues to use Tampax.   (S.V.M.)

Tassaway cups are more expensive than pads or tampons, and they are
not always comfortable once inserted. Furthermore, several women I
know who tried them said they sometimes were difficult to remove,
but this is information from a very small group and may not be the
average experience. If the expense is not too great for your budget,
cups are worth a try. This is especially true, I would think, for the
women who have complained about the problems with tampons.
Several women answering the questionnaire said that because their
jobs demand long hours outdoors away from toilet facilities, tampon
changing and disposal become a problem. Cups might solve both
problems. Women who do a lot of camping may also prefer cups,
since one is faced with less material to dispose of.

A new product needs to be developed, one that is inexpensive,
collects a large amount of flow, is easy to use, can be flushed down a
toilet (without causing a plumbing upheaval), and is worn internally.

As the women's movement has grown, more women have begun to
study aspects of female experience. Some of the results of this new
effort have been seen in the research reported in this book. Every
student of medicine, anthropology, behavior, endocrinology, or physiology will no doubt have her own hierarchy of relevant questions in
need of answers, as will every woman who thinks about the female

condition. The following is the list of important questions I discovered during the years in which I researched and wrote this book:

1. *Longitudinal studies*. Starting during puberty, if records were
maintained that included an individual's feelings about and physical
experiences with menstruation, pregnancy, postpartum response, premenopause, menopause, and the post-menopause, as well as all the
information found in ordinary medical histories, we could learn the
nature of normal experience in a woman's life, which stages of life
bear on others, and the ways in which our individual experience is
similar or different from that of other women.

2. *Menstrual and menopausal synchrony*. What, if they exist, are
the variables that result in menstrual and menopausal synchrony? If
this area were researched, we would have a stronger sense of the
important factors that influence the cycles of menstruation and
menopause.

3. *Birth control*. Researchers in the field of population control
have focused their attention on the "workability" of different
methods of birth control and the practical "problems" of having
people use contraception. The whole issue of possible side effects has
received comparatively little attention. But the research into the ways
contraceptives affect the menstrual cycle or menstrual symptoms has
been negligible. Very little is known about the ways in which the pill
alters premenstrual symptoms or how it affects the full range of cyclic
experience; even less is known about IUD's. It has been assumed that
women will tolerate virtually any menstrual upheaval in exchange for
effective contraception—and in many cases they have done so. While
we want safe and effective contraception, we should not accept the
idea that we are "cursed." And those who research and develop
contraceptive methods should less cavalierly promote products that
coincidentally create menstrual upheaval.

4. *Behavior and menstruation and menopause*. Those studies that
have dealt with behavior and the menstrual cycle have focused on the
disarray of the premenstrual phase, and those dealing with the behavioral aspects of menopause, on disability. Just as information on the
physical aspects of these cycles is needed, we would also benefit from
more information about behavioral changes that will follow only
when these studies are well designed, include large enough samples,
and cover the *full* range of behavior and experience.

Such studies must be combined with longitudinal surveys. As it
now stands, there are indications, trends, preliminary findings, and so

forth, but very little solid information about the relationship between the menstrual cycle or menopause and women's feelings and behavior. The little that has been done all too quickly becomes a part of the common knowledge of menstruation and menopause, but because it is not sufficiently solid data, it might more aptly be considered part of the folklore of menstruation. Mary Brown Parlee, in a review of the literature dealing with menstruation, concluded:

> Psychological studies of the premenstrual syndrome have not yet established the existence of a class of behaviors and moods measurable *in more than one way* which can be shown in a longitudinal study to fluctuate throughout the course of the menstrual cycle or even a class of such behaviors which is clearly correlated with any particular phase of the cycle for groups of women. This is not to say that such a set of behaviors does not exist—many women spontaneously attest that they do—but that as a scientific hypothesis the existence of premenstrual syndrome has little other than face validity.[4]

Researchers with an interest in women's issues have scores of projects ahead of them. It would be most instructive, for example, to have a series of studies on male behavior and menstruation (i.e., sexual response to menstruating women), as well as on male attitudes toward menstruation and menopause. Not the least interesting subcategory of this type of study would be an analysis of the attitudes held by physicians—particularly gynecologists.

5. *Physiology.* Almost every physical aspect of the menstrual cycle and the menopausal experience is poorly understood. It is clear that much more time and money needs to be devoted to these basic biological functions in order to understand how they normally function and what occurs in abnormal function. Parallel to this is the need to embark on a major research campaign in order to learn the ways in which malfunction may be successfully treated—without endangering women's health.

Women don't have to accept pain, discomfort, and the many side effects of hormonal change. Certainly, minor problems with menstruation and menopause can be endured; but when they are no longer exacerbated by negative cultural stereotypes, they may be less painful.

In recent years I have found that not all women consider menstrual blood disgusting. Some find it a confirmation of their femaleness— their potential to bear children—their inner self. This has helped me to change my attitudes—to at least accept it as a part of every month. . . . Another help has been my discovery that not all men view menstruation as repulsive—or sex as dirty. This makes me less inclined to conceal my cramps and/or feel ashamed of myself while I'm menstruating. That, too, eases the headaches and pain. (L.L.P.)

A certain amount of menstrual distress is caused by cultural attitude. However, we must take care not to mistake a part for the whole. Not all cases of menstrual or menopausal discomfort will be dramatically reduced or "cured" by changes in attitudes.

Painless menstruation or symptom-free menopause are sound goals for medical research, but they ought not to be moral ideals. Perfection of the female spirit will not cure all ills, whether perfection is defined by a gynecologist or a woman. Any woman who is suffering with menstrual or menopausal problems has the right to relief and cure of these discomforts, and such remedies must be rigorously sought after. A woman is not born to suffer (or overcome suffering through moral perfection) any more than she is born unclean. While there is plenty of evidence that women have remarkable capacities to endure pain, there is no evidence that we are born masochists or saints. Female masochism appears to be one more male fantasy rationalizing male inattention to women's needs, and female "bravery" appears to be the women's counterpart to the concept of masochism.

This list of research proposals is only the most meager beginning. As women start to become aware of the taboo, more and more questions will arise, and there will be greater demand to find the answers to these questions.

It is obvious that changes in our attitudes about menstruation and menopause must be passed on to coming generations of women and men. Many women who responded to the menstrual questionnaire are trying to provide the young with a better education than they were given.

I have told my daughters about menstruation: the older one (ten) seems accepting. The younger one (five) seems positively excited.

(S.G.)

I have two sons, aged thirteen and seven, and they have been informed about menstruation and are very accepting of their mother's monthly cycle. (M.J.W.)

Recently I was complaining to my fifteen-year-old sister about the cramps I was having. She referred to menstruation as the "Dirty Devil." I found myself getting mad and telling her, "There's nothing dirty or evil about it!" I felt oddly proud of this process, not because it was a burden but because it was natural and womanly. . . .

(M.J.W.)

. . . We have always had an open bathroom policy so they [the children] grew up fully observant of the fact that at times I had a bit more cleanup to perform than at other times. Eventually, one of them saw me actually remove a used tampon and said, "What's that?"

I told her what it was, where I got it, what it was used for and how I was going to dispose of it. She asked me if she would have to do that too someday. I said yes she would.

When the older daughter passed her twelfth birthday I placed a supply of sanitary napkins and a choice of belts and panties on a shelf in their closet, and told both girls that the supplies were there, and if they wanted to experiment ahead of time with brands to find which was most comfortable I would purchase any kind they wanted. (J.C.B.)

My children ages 3–8 years, girls and boys, are all aware of menstruation. They've seen me changing pads and tampons. They want it explained over and over again.   (L.J.)

We have two daughters, twelve and seven. The twelve-year-old has just had her first menstruation. . . . Her father and sister and I were able to share her first menstruation. We drank wine and toasted her. Her father gave her a bunch of wild flowers. She seemed pleased and open. She seems to identify positively with her sex. . . . Even though I was really unhappy and found my sex distasteful (for sixteen or seventeen years) my daughter appears relaxed and matter of fact with her sex and her physical changes. . . . It is a continual source of surprise and deep pleasure to me.   (C.C.B.)

In each case, teaching younger people to have a more open and accepting attitude implies that the adult has reassessed her early training.

Although some women—and men—are educating themselves, this is far from universal. Educational institutions and the people who rule them will have to assume the task of teaching the coming generations more adequately and more humanely. So far this job has not been done on any large scale.

A national survey of unmarried adolescent girls has indicated that, among the 2.4 million who have had sexual intercourse, more than half failed to use any form of contraception the last time they had sexual relations.

They also showed that teenagers who fail to use contraception often have as their reason their "belief that conception could not occur because sex was too infrequent, the girl was too young, or it was the 'wrong time of the month,' " Dr. Kantner and Dr. Zelnick reported.

An earlier finding showed that only about two-fifths of the teenagers surveyed know when in the menstrual cycle a woman is most likely to get pregnant.[5]

Some 5 million sexually active young women and men don't have adequate knowledge about the menstrual cycle, fertility, and contraception, and we can assume that millions more among the sexually less active share these areas of ignorance.

Girls and boys ought to learn about menstruation and menopause, not only because of the connection between fertility and menstruation. All the facts of life (cyclicity as well as fertility) are part of the lives women and men *share*. Yet this concept is lost on many members of the community.

I wanted to show the films on menstruation to the junior high boys. (I was willing to show it separately to just the boys, as a concession to the general horror expressed by the girls.) But I could not get permission from the local school board.

I am now a member of our school board but I am making no progress at all trying to convince my fellow members that sex education is not a communist plot, that boys need to know about menstruation and they should be properly informed about it, that pregnant girls should be allowed to attend school—I horrified the men at the last board meeting by reminding them that for every unwed mother there lurks somewhere in the background also an unwed father—and that girls and women in general should not have to apologize for being girls and women.

(A.M.H.)

As adults we suffer from deficient or warped education, and while some want to provide a better base for the next generations, there are others who create obstacles. Women's groups, for example, are perfectly free to offer courses on health in alternate institutions but access to the established educational channels is not easy. I was approached by an administrator at a university who asked me to teach a "consumer" course on women's health. (This institution, by the way, already offered many "women's" courses of a more academic sort.) The head of the university vetoed the course because I am not a physician. I tried to explain that if physicians were doing a good job of educating patients (good by women's standards) this course would be unnecessary. We went a few more rounds and the subject was "tabled." This administrator like many of his colleagues would do well to ponder the following words from Margaret Mead: "If we once accept the premise that we can build a better world by using the gifts of each sex, we shall have two kinds of freedom, freedom to use untapped gifts of each sex, and freedom to admit freely and cultivate in each sex their special superiorities."[6]

Part of the reason that needed changes (like research priorities) have not been made is that enough women have not demanded them and acted to get them. As long as we continue to accept the taboo, these changes will not be made, all our gifts not contributed, and we will remain submerged in our silence.

Recent history offers an example of the ways in which a lack of belief in the self can limit women's experience and possibility for expansion. During the so-called sexual revolution, women battled the double standard and in substantial degree refused to believe in it or act upon it any longer. However, as long as we believed that common knowledge and the "experts" on female sexuality were correct, that there were two separate kinds of orgasm—the clitoral and the "mature" vaginal—many "liberated" women believed themselves to be the walking wounded. Only when Masters and Johnson published their findings on orgasmic response did common knowledge conform with what women had been saying was their actual experience. For years we have been saying what we actually felt during sexual response—but because no one believed us, we often didn't believe ourselves. Perhaps the most demanding challenge in overthrowing taboo will come from within each of us as we start to believe what our bodies and feelings tell us.

As women come together, discover commonalities and differences, and articulate their needs, as they work on research questions of mutual concern and educate the coming generations, they will gain greater confidence in their individual experiences. It is well known by now that among the many issues confronting those who wish to build a world in which the next generations of women will have equality, those of sex are the most pernicious.

In order to move into the world that Mead describes, men and women must cooperate rather than compete. If one sex is hostile to the other, the object of hostility is believed to be dangerous and the bearer of hostility *is* dangerous. The menstrual taboo codifies sexual hostility and therefore gives evidence of the war between the sexes in our culture. Douglas, in describing the attitudes among the Lele, might well have been describing our own:

> Female pollution in a society of this type is largely related to the attempt to treat women simultaneously as persons and as the currency of male transactions. Males and females are set off as belonging to distinct, mutually hostile spheres. Sexual antagonism inevitably results and this is reflected in the idea that each sex represents a danger to the other. The particular dangers which female contact threatens to males express their contradiction of trying to use women as currency without reducing them to slavery. If ever it was felt in a culture that money is the root of all evil, the feeling that women are the root of all evils to Lele men is even more justified. Indeed the story of the Garden of Eden touched a deep chord of sympathy in Lele male breasts. Once told by the missionaries, it was told and retold round the pagan hearths with smug relish.[7]

Obviously, competition between the sexes reflects the competition within the sexes. Males, using females as currency, fight among each other to be the richest and most powerful, while women fight among one another to be possessed by the richest and most powerful.

As women have questioned societal beliefs, we have re-examined the competition between members of our own sex. It would be delusional to say this problem has been solved, but it is realistic to say it has changed somewhat. We have begun to make the necessary alterations so that the competitive system and the taboo which underlies it can be challenged. To quote Mead again, "Once it is possible to say it is as important to take woman's gifts and make them available to both men and women, in transmittable form, as it was to take men's gifts and make the civilization built upon them available to both men and women, we shall have enriched our society."[8] As the taboo disintegrates, so will the hostility between the sexes which it both reflects and feeds. The witch doctor will turn in his bag of tricks, the analyst his blindfold, and the rank and file their fear that their sex will lose all its powers if women are no longer defined by men.

There are an unending number of provisions in the plan to dismantle the taboo which are subject to direct actions and forms of legislation. But the menstrual taboo is an outgrowth of sexual combat, sexual antagonisms keep it alive, and in this arena the deepest as well as the darkest of human feelings dwell.

For many of us, danger is wedded to sexual attraction. For man, woman is dangerous because she menstruates—the mystery and power which may harm him. She is no longer as sexually attractive when menstruation ceases. For woman, man is dangerous because of his worldly powers; this is his sexual attraction—he has the potential for overpowering. For each sex there is the danger of annihilation and the sexual charge of that risk.

It is time for women to reclaim menstruation and menopause. Each day one of these cycles is part of our lives; yet we live with a male idea of how we ought to feel about them. We may clasp the earth mother to our breasts and proclaim the beauty of menopause and the marvel of menstruation, but this is no more necessary than hanging on to the witch who bears a curse. Somewhere between the goddess and the demon is the menstruating woman and after her the woman at menopause—living women with cycles of life not experienced by men, different and equal.

Appendix: The Questionnaire

Notes

Selected Bibliography

Appendix: The Questionnaire

I am writing a book about menstruation, menopause, and puberty. As you know, there's little information on these subjects that is now available. I want the book to be useful and meet the readers' needs and so have put together this questionnaire. Please feel that you can answer any of the questions more fully than space allotted indicates and add anything you feel is relevant. Thanks for your help.

By what term do you refer to menstruation?

At what age did you begin to menstruate?

How did you first learn about it?

When you began to menstruate, did you feel you had been adequately prepared? yes___, no___. If no, what might have helped you?

When you learned about menstruation, did you know "how babies are made"? yes___, no___. Did you understand the relationship between sex and reproduction? yes___, no___, sort of___.

Did your attitude toward boys change when you began to menstruate? yes___, no___. If yes, how?

Did your attitude toward yourself change? yes___, no___. If yes, how?

Was your first flow a positive experience___, negative___, neutral___, frightening___, exciting___?

Are you aware of any physical or emotional changes during the menstrual cycle? yes___, no___. If yes, when do they occur and what are they?

Have you found any successful method of dealing with menstrual cramps or other forms of menstrual distress? If yes, what?

What "old wives' tales" or home remedies were passed on to you about menstruation?

Is there a particular time of the month when you feel sexually turned on? yes___, no___. If yes, when?

Have partners objected to sexual activity when you are menstruating? yes___, no___, occasionally___. Do you object to sex when you're menstruating? yes___, no___. If yes, why?

At what time of the month is conception most likely to occur?

Is there a time of the month when it is impossible to conceive?

What form of birth control do you use___, and does it affect your menstrual cycle experience or flow? yes___, no___. If yes, how?

If you could retain fertility but have no more menstrual flow would you opt for that? yes___, no___. Why?

Is there anything you would like to know about menstruation? About menopause?

How many years have you been menstruating?

Do you feel that menstruation brings any special advantage to women? yes___, no___. If yes, what?

Do you feel that men have special advantage because they do *not* menstruate? yes___, no___. If yes, what?

What is your religious background?

The intention of this questionnaire was exactly as stated. I did not set out to do a study of menstrual attitudes; rather, I wanted to give women an opportunity to share their experience and feelings. (There was a separate questionnaire for menopause and one to be answered by men. These have not been reproduced because the number of people to whom they were distributed and from whom they were returned was small.)

The questionnaires were distributed in the following way: Ms. magazine provided me with space in the personal column in the spring of 1973. In the ad I said I was writing a book about menstruation and menopause, that I had prepared a questionnaire, and asked people to write to me in care of my publisher if they wished to help with the preparation of the book by giving their views.

Although I had been told to expect a large response, I was completely unprepared for the volume of mail I received. More than 1,000 women wrote to ask for the questionnaire and, of this group, 500 asked for a copy also of the questionnaire for men. Almost 600 women (of whom 558 completely filled out the form) then returned the questionnaires.

While I did not do an analysis of the geographical distribution of requests and replies, I did read each request and every returned questionnaire and can report that those who answered were not clustered in any major city, nor were they concentrated in the coastal regions. They literally came from all over the United States, from across Canada, and from scattered outposts throughout the world. (I received at least one response each from Japan, Mexico, Puerto Rico, Guam, Okinawa, as well as from a number of European countries.)

Age of women at the time they answered the questions:
Sixteen percent of the women responding were below the age of twenty (the youngest was twelve); 58 percent were between twenty and thirty; 17 percent between thirty and forty; and 8 percent between forty and fifty-eight (the oldest was fifty-eight).

Age at menarche:
Two women reported the start of menstruation in the year following their eighth birthday; ten said they began their ninth birthday; thirty-nine after their tenth. Seventy-five percent said they came to menarche between their eleventh and fourteenth birthdays (102 women at eleven, 155 at twelve, and 161 at thirteen). Following the fourteenth birthday, fifty-seven began menstruating; after the fifteenth, nineteen began. Ten women started menstruating after age sixteen, two after seventeen, and one after eighteen.

Religion:
Forty-two percent of the women were raised in Protestant homes, 30 percent in Catholic homes, and 16 percent in Jewish homes. Seventy-two percent currently practice (in some fashion) the religion in which they were raised.

As I have said, I did not intend this to be a behavioral study. However, when presented with the amount of information that was sent to me and the size of the response, it became increasingly apparent that use of this material should not be confined to this book.

For these reasons, the data have been made available to a graduate student in psychology, Ann Litwin, who, with the permission of the women involved, will acquire more demographic information and continue an analysis of responses as part of her master's thesis.

Notes

1 VEILS AND VARIABILITY

1. Alan E. Treolar *et al.*, "Variations of Human Menstrual Cycle through Reproductive Life," *Internat. J. Fertility* 12:77, 1967. p. 81.
2. H. R. Hays, *The Dangerous Sex* (New York: Pocket Books, 1972), p. 33.
3. C. D. Daly, "The Role of Menstruation in Human Phylogenesis and Ontogenesis," *Internat. J. Psychoanal.* 24:151, 1943. p. 169.
4. R. V. Cassill, *The Goss Women* (New York: Doubleday and Company, 1974), p. 380.

2 THE MENSTRUAL CYCLE

1. J. M. Tanner, *Growth at Adolescence* (2nd ed. Springfield, Ill.: Charles C Thomas, 1962).
2. In a series of papers Dr. Frisch (in some cases joined by Dr. Roger Revelle) has published the findings leading to the conclusions on critical weight. Of these I have relied most on Frisch, "Critical Weights, a Critical Body Composition, Menarche and the Maintenance of Menstrual Cycles," in *Biosocial Interrelation in Population Adaptation.* Mouton & Co., The Hague. (In press.)
3. W. H. Masters and V. E. Johnson, *Human Sexual Response* (Boston: Little, Brown and Company, 1966).
4. S. Leon Israel, *Menstrual Disorders and Sterility* (5th ed. New York: Harper & Row, 1967), p. 101.
5. L. Chiazze, Jr., *et al.*, "The Length and Variability of the Human Menstrual Cycle," *JAMA*, Vol. 203, No. 6. February 5, 1968. pp. 89–92.
6. Flora L. Bailey, "Some Sex Beliefs and Practices in a Navaho Community," *Papers of the Peabody Museum of American Archaeology and Ethnology*, Harvard University, Vol. XL, No. 2, Cambridge, Mass., 1950.
7. Martha K. McClintock, "Menstrual Synchrony and Suppression," *Nature*, Vol. 229, No. 5282, January 1971. pp. 244–5.
8. *Ibid.*
9. Rodrigo Guerrero, "Association of the Type and Time of Insemination within the Menstrual Cycle with the Human Sex Ratio at Birth," *New Engl. J. Med.*, 291:20, November 1974. p. 1056.

10. Barbara Seaman, *The Doctors' Case Against the Pill* (New York: Avon Books, 1970), p. 121.

3 "COMPLAINTS," CAUSES AND CURES

1. Virginia Scully, *Treasury of American Indian Herbs* (New York: Crown Publishing Company, 1970).
2. Oscar Janiger, Ralph Riffenburgh, and Ronald Kersh, "Cross Cultural Study of Premenstrual Symptoms," *Psychosomatics*, Vol. 13, July–August 1972. p. 232.
3. B. P. Appleby, "A Study of Premenstrual Tension in General Practice." *Brit. Med. J.* 1:391. February 1960.
4. Katharina Dalton, *The Menstrual Cycle* (New York: Pantheon Books, 1969), p. 55. In this book, Dr. Dalton summarizes her findings concerning premenstrual syndrome and her theories about its origin.
5. J. F. O'Connor, E. M. Shelley, and Lenore O. Stern, "Behavioral Rhythms Related to the Menstrual Cycle," *International Institute for the Study of Human Reproduction*. New York, 1973. p. 7.
6. Richard I. Shader and Jane I. Ohly, "Premenstrual Tension, Femininity, and Sexual Drive," *Medical Aspects of Human Sexuality*, April 1970. p. 48.
7. Sakari Timonen and Berndt-Johan Procopé, "Premenstrual Syndrome and Physical Exercise," *Acta Obstet. Gynecol. Scan.* 50:333–7, 1971.
8. *Ibid.*, p. 336.
9. Dalton, *op. cit.*, p. 62.
10. Personal communication.
11. Joseph Gilman, "Nature of Subjective Reaction Evoked in Women by Progesterone with Special Reference to the Problem of Premenstrual Tension." *J. Clin. Endocrin.* 2:156, 1942.
12. Dalton, *op. cit.*, p. 61.
13. G. W. Thorne, "Cyclical Edema," *Am. J. Med.* 23:507, 1957.
14. Lena Levine and Beka Doherty, *The Menopause* (New York: Random House, 1952), pp. 5–6.
15. J. Money and A. A. Ehrhardt, *Man, Woman, Boy, Girl* (Baltimore, Md.: Johns Hopkins University Press, 1972), pp. 223–4.
16. S. Leon Israel, *Diagnosis and Treatment of Menstrual Disorders and Sterility* (5th ed. New York: Harper & Row, 1967), p. 398.
17. Herbert S. Kupperman, "The Climacteric Syndrome," *The Medical Folio.* 5:1, 1972. p. 1.
18. Robert A. Wilson, *Feminine Forever* (New York: M. Evans and Company, 1966), p. 79.
19. Kupperman, *op. cit.*, p. 2.
20. Dalton, *op. cit.*, p. 42.
21. Jane E. Brody, "Pain Killer Test Is Led by Aspirin," *New York Times*, March 1, 1972. p. 13.
22. Israel, *op. cit.*, pp. 363–4.

4 TABOO

1. H. R. Hays, *The Dangerous Sex* (New York: Pocket Books, 1972).
2. Pliny, *Natural History*, Vol. VII, p. 15.
3. *Ibid.*, Vol. XXVIII, p. 23.
4. Hays, *op. cit.*, p. 30.
5. James Frazer, *The New Golden Bough*, edited by Theodore Gaster (New York: New American Library, 1959), pp. 212–13.

6. Hays, *op. cit.*, pp. 30–1.
7. Raymond Crawfurd, "Superstitions of Menstruation," *The Lancet*, December 18, 1915. p. 1333.
8. Emil Novak, *Menstruation and Its Disorders* (New York: D. Appleton and Company, 1921), p. 3.
9. Crawfurd, *op. cit.*, p. 1333.
10. Novak, *op. cit.*, p. 3.
11. H. H. Ploss, M. Bartles, and P. Bartles, *Woman: An Historical, Gynecological and Anthropological Compendium*; edited by E. J. Dingwall (London: William Heinemann Ltd., 1935), Vol. III, p. 408. Quotes appearing later in this chapter from Vol. I are freely translated from the original German edition published by Neufeld & Henius Verlag, Berlin, 1927.
12. Frazer, *op. cit.*, pp. 210–11.
13. William N. Stevens, "A Cross-cultural Study of Menstrual Taboos," In *Cross-cultural Approaches*, edited by Clellan S. Ford (New Haven, Conn.: HRAF Press, 1967), p. 75.
14. Ploss and Bartles, *op. cit.*, Vol. I.
15. Crawfurd, *op. cit.*, p. 1331.
16. *Ibid.*
17. "All in the Family," Tandem Productions. Written by Michael Ross and Bernie West. Copyright © 1973.
18. Sigmund Freud, "The Taboo of Virginity," in *The Case of Dora and Other Papers* (New York: W. W. Norton & Company, 1952), p. 231.
19. Personal communication.
20. Frazer, *op. cit.*, pp. 224–5.
21. Freud, *op. cit.*, p. 229.
22. Hays, *op. cit.*, pp. 29–30.
23. Daly, *op. cit.*, p. 164.
24. Sigmund Freud, *Totem and Taboo*, translated by James Strachery (New York: W. W. Norton & Company, 1950), p. 144.
25. Goethe, quoted by Freud, *Totem and Taboo*, p. 161.
26. Ploss and Bartles, *op. cit.*, pp. 783–4.
27. Freud, "The Taboo of Virginity," *op. cit.*, pp. 242–3.
28. Daly, *op. cit.*, p. 163.
29. Gerardo Reichel-Dolmatoff, *Amazonian Cosmos* (Chicago & London: The University of Chicago Press, 1971), pp. 28–9.
30. Daly, *op. cit.*, p. 163.
31. Juliet Mitchell, *Psychoanalysis and Feminism* (New York: Pantheon Books, 1974), p. 406.
32. Frazer, *op. cit.*, p. 360.
33. Frieda Fromm-Reichmann and Virginia K. Gunst, "On the Denial of Women's Sexual Pleasure," in *Psychoanalysis and Women*, edited by Jean Baker Miller (Baltimore, Md.: Penguin Books, 1973), p. 88.
34. Bruno Bettelheim, *Symbolic Wounds* (New York: Collier Books, 1962), p. 123.
35. *Ibid.*, p. 129.
36. *Ibid.*, p. 100, quoting B. Spencer and F. J. Gillen, *The Native Tribes of Central Australia* (London: Macmillan & Co., 1899), pp. 255–7.
37. *Ibid.*, p. 105.
38. G. Devereux, "The Psychology of Feminine Genital Bleeding," *Intern. J. Psychoanal.*, Vol. XXXI, 1950. p. 252.
39. Mary Jane Sherfey, "On the Nature of Female Sexuality," in *Psychoanalysis and Women*, p. 151.

40. *Ibid.*, p. 151.
41. Ploss and Bartles, *op. cit.*, p. 784.
42. Mary Chadwick, *The Psychology of Menstruation* (Monograph 56) (Washington, D.C.: Nervous and Mental Diseases Publishing Company, 1932), p. 11.
43. *Ibid.*, p. 18.
44. Lester Ward, quoted by Gregory Zilboorg, "Masculine and Feminine: Some Biological and Cultural Aspects," in *Psychoanalysis and Women*, p. 114.
45. *Ibid.*, p. 128.
46. *Ibid.*, p. 119.
47. Fromm-Reichmann and Gunst, *op. cit.*, p. 88.

5 THE SEXUAL CYCLE

1. Raymond Crawfurd, "Superstitions of Menstruation," *The Lancet*, December 18, 1915. p. 1335.
2. Karen Paige, "Women Learn to Sing the Menstrual Blues," *Psychology Today*, September 1973.
3. J. M. Bardwick and J. Zweben, reported in Judith M. Bardwick, *Psychology of Women* (New York: Harper & Row, 1971), pp. 54–5.
4. Mary Jane Sherfey, *The Nature and Evolution of Female Sexuality* (New York: Random House, 1972), pp. 98–9.
5. T. Benedek and B. B. Rubenstein, "The Sexual Cycle in Women," *Psychosomatic Med. Monographs* (Washington, D.C.: National Research Council, 1942), 3, Nos. 1 and 2.
6. T. Benedek, *Studies in Psychosomatic Medicine: Psychosexual Functions* (New York: The Ronald Press Company, 1952), pp. 144–8.
7. Alfred C. Kinsey *et al.*, *Sexual Behavior in the Human Female* (New York: Pocket Books, 1970).
8. J. R. Udry and N. Morris, "Distribution of Coitus in the Menstrual Cycle," *Nature* (London). 220:593, November 1968.
9. M. Esther Harding, *Woman's Mysteries* (New York: Bantam Books, 1973), pp. 92–3.
10. Crawfurd, *op. cit.*, p. 1334.

6 WITCH DOCTORS

1. Claude Lévi-Strauss, "The Sorcerer and His Magic," in *Structural Anthropology*, translated by Claire Jacobsen and Brooke Grundfest Schoepf (New York: Basic Books, 1963).
2. W. S. Kroger, *Psychosomatic Obstetrics, Gynecology and Endocrinology* (Springfield, Ill.: Charles C Thomas, Publisher, 1962), p. 257.
3. Sherwin A. Kaufman, *The Ageless Woman* (Englewood Cliffs, N.J.: Prentice-Hall, Inc., 1967), pp. 20–1.
4. Diana Scully and Pauline Bart, "A Funny Thing Happened on the Way to the Orifice," *Amer. J. Sociol.*, 78:4, January 1973. pp. 1045–50.
5. Boston Women's Health Collective, *Our Bodies, Our Selves* (New York: Simon and Schuster, 1973), p. 251.
6. Helene Deutsch, *The Psychology of Women* (New York: Grune and Stratton, 1944), Vol I., pp. 166–7.
7. K. Jean Lennane and R. John Lennane, "Alleged Psychogenic Disorders in Women—A Possible Manifestation of Sexual Prejudice," *New Engl. J. Med.*, February 8, 1973. pp. 288–92.

8. Constance Berry and Frederick L. McGuire, "Menstrual Distress and Acceptance of Sexual Role," *Am. J. Obstet. Gynecol.*, 114:1, September 1, 1972. p. 84.

9. *Ibid.*

10. *Ibid.*, p. 86.

11. Virginia Woolf, *A Room of One's Own* (New York: Harcourt, Brace & World, 1957), pp. 113–14.

12. Lévi-Strauss, *op. cit.*, p. 168.

13. Sonja M. McKinlay and John B. McKinlay, "Selected Studies of the Menopause," *J. Biosoc. Sci.* 5, 1973. p. 535.

14. Alice James, Diary excerpted in *Revelations: Diaries of Women*, edited by Mary Jane Moffat and Charlotte Painter (New York: Random House, 1974), p. 199.

15. Lennane and Lennane, *op. cit.*, p. 291.

16. Ruth Benedict, Diary excerpted in *Revelations, op. cit.*, pp. 150–1.

17. Boston Women's Health Collective, *op. cit.*, p. 253.

18. Phyllis Chesler, *Women and Madness* (New York: Doubleday and Company, 1972), p. 243.

19. Virginia Woolf, *Three Guineas* (New York: Harcourt, Brace & World, 1963), pp. 181–7 (f. 32).

7 TODAY YOU ARE A WOMAN

1. Quarinonius, *Die Grewel der Verwürslung menschlichen Geschleckts.* Innsbruck, 1610. Quoted in L. Zacharias and R. J. Wurtman, "Age at Menarche," *New Engl. J. Med.* 280:16, April 17, 1969. p. 873. Modern-day research on critical weight is reported in chapters 2 and 3.

2. Margaret Mead, *Sex and Temperament* (New York: William Morrow & Company, 1935), pp. 92–3.

3. H. S. Arnstein, *Your Growing Child and Sex* (New York: Avon Books, 1967), p. 133.

4. Judith M. Bardwick, *Psychology of Women* (New York: Harper & Row, 1971), p. 13.

5. Helene Deutsch, *The Psychology of Women* (New York: Grune and Stratton, 1944), Vol. I, p. 156.

6. Simone de Beauvoir, *The Second Sex* (Harmondsworth, Middlesex: Penguin Books, 1972), p. 180.

7. Deutsch, *op. cit.*, p. 152.

8. Grace Paley, "Faith in the Afternoon," in *Enormous Changes at the Last Minute* (New York: Farrar, Straus & Giroux, 1974), p. 44.

9. M. F. Ashley Montagu, *The Reproductive Development of the Female with Especial Reference to the Period of Adolescent Sterility* (New York: Julian Press, 1957).

10. De Beauvoir, *op. cit.*, p. 340.

11. Tennessee Williams, "The Resemblance Between a Violin Case and a Coffin," in *Hard Candy: A Book of Stories* (New York: New Directions, 1954), pp. 81–4.

12. Elizabeth Douvan, "New Sources of Conflict in Females at Adolescence and Early Adulthood," in *Feminine Personality and Conflict* (Belmont, Calif.: Brooks/Cole Publishing Co., 1970), p. 32.

13. Katharina Dalton, *The Menstrual Cycle* (New York: Pantheon Books, 1969).

14. Douvan, *op. cit.*, p. 33.

15. J. C. Webster, *Puberty and the Change of Life* (Edinburgh: E. & S. Livingstone, 1892).
16. George Gilder, "Sexual Suicide," *Harper's*, July 1973. p. 49.
17. M. F. Ashley Montagu, *The Natural Superiority of Women* (New York: The Macmillan Company, 1953), p. 33.
18. Clara Thompson, "Cultural Pressures in the Psychology of Women," in *Psychoanalysis and Women*, edited by Jean Baker Miller (Baltimore, Md.: Pelican Books, 1973), pp. 74–5.

8 WOMAN IN THE MOON

1. M. Esther Harding, *Woman's Mysteries* (New York: Bantam Books, 1973), pp. 78–9.
2. *Ibid.*, p. 75.
3. Alfred Tafel, *Meine Tibetreise* (Stuttgart: Union Deutsche Verlag, 1914), Vol. II, pp. 332–3.
4. Margaret Mead, *Sex and Temperament* (New York: William Morrow & Company, 1935), p. 70.
5. Georg Simmel, quoted by Karen Horney in "The Flight from Womanhood," in *Psychoanalysis and Women*, edited by Jean Baker Miller (Baltimore, Md.: Penguin Books, 1973), p. 6.
6. Virginia Woolf, *A Room of One's Own* (New York: Harcourt, Brace & World, 1957), p. 108.
7. *Ibid.*
8. Cynthia Ozick, "The Demise of the Dancing Dog," in *Women in Sexist Society*, edited by Vivian Gornick and Barbara K. Moran (New York: New American Library, 1972), p. 439.
9. Melville E. Ivey and Judith M. Bardwick, "Patterns of Affective Fluctuation in the Menstrual Cycle," reported in J. M. Bardwick, *Psychology of Women* (New York: Harper & Row, 1971), pp. 31–2.
10. Bardwick, *Psychology of Women*, p. 32.
11. Katharina Dalton, *The Menstrual Cycle* (New York: Pantheon Books, 1969).
12. P. C. B. MacKinnon and I. L. MacKinnon, "Hazards of the Menstrual Cycle," *Brit. Med. J.* 1:555, 1956.
13. R. D. Wetzel and J. N. McClure, Jr., "Suicide and the Menstrual Cycle: A Review," *Comprehensive Psychiatry*. 13:4, 1972. pp. 369–74.
14. P. de Ondegardo, "Information on the Religion of the Incas," Research carried out in 1916, HRAF Files, 1965.
15. Havelock Ellis, *Sexual Periodicity* (Chicago, Ill.: Behavior Classics).
16. Karen Paige, "Women Learn to Sing the Menstrual Blues," *Psychology Today*, September 1973. pp. 41–6.
17. *Ibid.*, p. 46.
18. Harding, *op. cit.*, pp. 93–4.

9 UNVEILED AND INVISIBLE

1. Margaret Mead, *Male and Female* (New York: Dell Publishing Company, 1970), p. 348.
2. Lena Levine and Beka Doherty, *The Menopause* (New York: Random House, 1952), pp. 49–50.
3. Bernice L. Neugarten and Ruth J. Kraines, " 'Menopausal Symptoms' in Women of Various Ages," *Psychosom. Med.* 27:3, 1965. pp. 266–73.
4. *Ibid.*, p. 272.

5. *Ibid.*
6. Sonja M. McKinlay and Margot Jefferys, "The Menopausal Syndrome," *Brit. J. Prev. and Soc. Med.* 28:2, 1974. pp. 108–15.
7. Sonja M. McKinlay and John B. McKinlay, "Selected Studies of the Menopause," *J. Biosoc. Sci.* 5, 1973. pp. 533–55.
8. Pauline Bart, "Depression in Middle-Aged Women," in *Women in Sexist Society*, edited by Vivian Gornick and Barbara K. Moran (New York: New American Library, 1972).
9. *Ibid.*, pp. 177–8.
10. *Ibid.*, p. 178.
11. *Ibid.*, p. 183.
12. *Ibid.*, p. 179.
13. Mead, *op. cit.*, p. 187.
14. M. J. Levy, *The Family Revolution in Modern China* (Cambridge, Mass.: Harvard University Press, 1948), p. 16.
15. Clara Thompson, *On Women* (New York: New American Library, 1971), p. 29.
16. H. H. Ploss, M. Bartles, and P. Bartles, *Woman: An Historical, Gynecological and Anthropological Compendium*, edited by E. J. Dingwall (London: William Heinemann Ltd., 1935), Vol. III.
17. Eckharth der Getrue, pseud. (J. C. Ettner), quoted in Ploss and Bartles, *op. cit.*, Vol. III, p. 347.
18. Arturo Vivanti, *Dr. Giovanni* (Boston: Little, Brown and Company, 1969), p. 75.
19. S. Leon Israel, *Menstrual Disorders and Sterility* (5th ed. New York: Harper & Row, 1967), p. 398.
20. Thompson, *op. cit.*, p. 171.
21. Vivian Gornick, *In Search of Ali Mahmoud* (New York: Saturday Review Press, 1973), pp. 70–1.
22. Doris Lessing, *The Summer Before the Dark* (New York: Alfred A. Knopf, 1973), pp. 22–3.
23. *Ibid.*, pp. 197–8.
24. Helene Deutsch, *The Psychology of Women* (New York: Grune and Stratton, 1944), Vol. II, pp. 459, 461.
25. Simone de Beauvoir, *The Second Sex* (Harmondsworth, Middlesex: Penguin Books, 1972), p. 588.
26. Deutsch, *op. cit.*, p. 477.
27. De Beauvoir, *op. cit.*, pp. 603–4.

10 CHANGES

1. Mary Douglas, *Purity and Danger: An Analysis of Concepts of Pollution and Taboo* (Baltimore, Md.: Penguin Books, 1970), p. 179.
2. Virginia Woolf, *A Room of One's Own* (New York: Harcourt, Brace & World, 1957), pp. 91–2.
3. Margaret Mead, *Male and Female* (New York: Dell Publishing Company, 1970), p. 358.
4. Mary Brown Parlee, "The Premenstrual Syndrome," *Psych. Bull.* 80:6, December 1973. p. 454.
5. Jane E. Brody, *New York Times*, March 1, 1973.
6. Mead, *op. cit.*, p. 358.
7. Douglas, *op. cit.*, pp. 180–1.
8. Mead, *op. cit.*, p. 358.

Selected Bibliography

Appleby, B. P. "A Study of Premenstrual Tension in General Practice," *British Medical Journal*, 1 (February 1960), 391.

Baden, W. F., and Lizcana, H. R. "Evaluation of a New Diuretic Drug (Quinethazon) in the Premenstrual Tension Syndrome," *Journal of New Drugs*, 3 (1963), 167.

Bailey, Flora L. "Some Sex Beliefs and Practices in a Navaho Community" (*Papers of the Peabody Museum of American Archaeology and Ethnology*, Harvard University, Vol. XL, No. 2), Cambridge, Mass., 1950.

Bardwick, Judith M. *Psychology of Women*. New York: Harper & Row, 1971.

Barnes, Allan C. "When Was Your Last Menstrual Period?" *Obstetrics and Gynecology*, 2 (1953), 664.

Bart, Pauline B. "Depression in Middle-aged Women," in *Women in Sexist Society*, Vivian Gornick and Barbara K. Moran (eds.). New York: New American Library, 1972.

———. "The Sociology of the Middle Years," *Sociological Symposium*, No. 3 (Fall 1969).

Beller, Fritz K. "Observations on the Clotting of Menstrual Blood," *American Journal of Obstetrics and Gynecology*, 111 (1971), 535.

Benedek, Therese. *Studies in Psychosomatic Medicine: Psychosexual Functions*. New York: The Ronald Press Company, 1952.

Benedek, Therese, and Rubenstein, B. B. "The Sexual Cycle in Women" (*Psychosomatic Medical Monographs*, 3, Nos. 1 and 2), Washington, D.C.: National Research Council, 1942.

Berry, Constance, and McGuire, Frederick L. "Menstrual Distress and Acceptance of Sexual Role," *American Journal of Obstetrics and Gynecology*, 114 (September 1972), 84.

Bettelheim, Bruno. *Symbolic Wounds*. New York: Collier Books, 1962.

Biskind, Leonard H., and Biskind, John I. "Functional Uterine Bleeding," *Missouri Medicine*, 3 (1956), 843.

Boston Women's Health Collective. *Our Bodies, Our Selves*. New York: Simon and Schuster, 1973.

Chadwick, Mary. *The Psychology of Menstruation* (Monograph 56). Washington, D.C.: Nervous and Mental Diseases Publishing Company, 1932.

Cherniak, Donna, and Feingold, Allan. *Birth Control Handbook*. Montréal: Montréal Health Press—Les Presses de la Santé de Montréal, Inc., 1973.

Chiazze, L., Jr., *et al.* "The Length and Variability of the Human Menstrual Cycle," *Journal of the American Medical Association*, 203:6 (1968).

Clark, Linda. "For Women Only," *Let's Live* (August 1970), 56.

Crawfurd, Raymond. "Superstitions of Menstruation," *The Lancet* (December 18, 1915).

Dalton, Katharina. *The Menstrual Cycle*. New York: Pantheon Books, 1969.

——. "Menstruation and Examinations," *The Lancet* (December 28, 1968), 1386.

——. "Schoolgirl's Behaviour and Menstruation," *British Medical Journal*, 2 (December 1960), 1647.

Daly, C. D. "The Role of Menstruation in Human Phylogenesis and Ontogenesis," *International Journal of Psychoanalysis*, 24 (1943), 151.

Davis, Adelle. *Let's Get Well*. New York: Harcourt, Brace & World, 1965.

De Beauvoir, Simone. *The Second Sex*. Harmondsworth, Middlesex: Penguin Books, 1972.

Deutsch, Helene. *The Psychology of Women*. Vols. I and II. New York: Grune and Stratton, 1944.

Devereux, G. "The Psychology of Feminine Genital Bleeding," *International Journal of Psychoanalysis, XXXI* (1950), 252.

Douglas, Mary. *Purity and Danger: An Analysis of Concepts of Pollution and Taboo*. Baltimore, Md.: Penguin Books, 1970.

Douvan, Elizabeth. "New Sources of Conflict in Females at Adolescence and Early Adulthood," in *Feminine Personality and Conflict*. Belmont, Calif.: Brooks/Cole Publishing Company, 1970.

Dunn, James. "Vicarious Menstruation," *American Journal of Obstetrics and Gynecology*, 114:4 (1972), 568.

Eichner, E., and Waltner, C. "Premenstrual Tension," *Medical Times*, 83 (1955), 771.

Ellis, Havelock. *Sexual Periodicity*. Chicago, Ill.: Behavior Classics.

Ford, Clellan S., and Beach, Frank A. *Patterns of Sexual Behavior*. New York: Perennial Library, Harper & Row, 1951.

Frank, R. T. "Hormonal Causes of Premenstrual Tension," *Archives of Neurology and Psychiatry*, 26 (1931), 1053.

Frazer, James. *The New Golden Bough*, Theodor Gaster (ed.). New York: New American Library, 1959.

Freud, Sigmund. *The Case of Dora and Other Papers*. New York: W. W. Norton & Company, 1952.

——. *New Introductory Lectures in Psychoanalysis*, translated by E. J. H. Sprott. New York: W. W. Norton & Company, 1933.

——. *Totem and Taboo*. Harmondsworth, Middlesex: Penguin Books, 1938.

Frisch, Rose E. "Critical Weights, a Critical Body Composition, Menarche and the Maintenance of Menstrual Cycles," in *Biosocial Interrelation in Population Adaptation*. The Hague: Mouton & Company. (In press.)

Frisch, Rose E., and Revelle, Roger. "Height and Weight at Menarche and a Hypothesis of Menarche," *Archives of Diseases in Childhood*, 46:249 (1971), 695.

Frisch, Rose E., Revelle, Roger, and Cook, Sole. "Components of Weight at

Menarche and the Initiation of the Adolescent Growth Spurt in Girls," *Human Biology*, 45:3 (1973), 169.

Gallagher, J. R. "Some Effects of Normal Endocrine Changes in Adolescence," *Postgraduate Medicine*, 34 (1963), 286.

Gilman, Joseph. "Nature of Subjective Reaction Evoked in Women by Progesterone with Special Reference to the Problem of Premenstrual Tension," *Journal of Clinical Endocrinology*, 2 (1942), 156.

Gottshalk, Louis A., *et al.* "Variation in Magnitude of Emotion: A Method Applied to Anxiety and Hostility During Phases of the Menstrual Cycle," *Psychosomatic Medicine*, 24 (1962), 300.

Greenblatt, Robert B. "Estrogen Therapy for Postmenopausal Females," *New England Journal of Medicine*, 272 (1963), 305.

Hamburg, David A. "Effects of Progesterone on Behavior," in Levine, Rachkiel (ed.), *Endocrines and the Central Nervous System*. Baltimore, Md.: Williams & Wilkins Company, 1966.

Hamburg, David A., and Lunde, Donald T. "Sex Hormones in the Development of Sex Differences in Human Behavior," in *The Development of Sex Differences*, Eleanor E. Maccoby (ed.). Stanford, Calif.: Stanford University Press, 1966.

Harding, M. Esther. *Woman's Mysteries*. New York: Bantam Books, 1973.

Hart, Ruth Darcy. "Monthly Rhythm of Libido in Married Women," *British Medical Journal*, 1 (1960), 1023.

Hays, H. R. *The Dangerous Sex*. New York: Pocket Books, 1972.

Israel, S. Leon. *Diagnosis and Treatment of Menstrual Disorders and Sterility*. Fifth edition, New York: Harper & Row, 1967.

Janiger, Oscar, Riffenburgh, Ralph, and Ronald Kersh. "Cross Cultural Study of Premenstrual Symptoms," *Psychosomatics*, 13 (1972), 226.

Janowsky, David S., Gorney, Roderick, and Kelley, Bret. " 'The Curse'—Vicissitudes and Variations of the Female Fertility Cycle," *Psychosomatics*, VII (1966), 242.

Johansson, E. D. B., Larsson-Cohn, U., and Gemzell, C. "Ovulatory Menstrual Cycles," *American Journal of Obstetrics and Gynecology*, 51 (1972), 77.

Jordheim, Odd. "The Premenstrual Syndrome," *Acta Obstetrica Gynecologica Scandinavica*, 51 (1972), 77.

Kaufman, Sherwin A. *The Ageless Woman*. Englewood Cliffs, N.J.: Prentice-Hall, 1967.

Kinsey, Alfred C., *et al.* *Sexual Behavior in the Human Female*. New York: Pocket Books, 1970.

Kleegman, Sophia J., and Kaufman, Sherwin A. "The Endocrines Concerned with Menstruation and Infertility," in *Infertility in Women*. Philadelphia: F. A. Davis, 1966.

Kroger, W. S. *Psychosomatic Obstetrics, Gynecology and Endocrinology*. Springfield, Ill.: Charles C Thomas, Publisher, 1962.

Kupperman, Herbert S. "The Climacteric Syndrome," *The Medical Folio*, 5 (1972).

Lennane, K. Jean, and Lennane, R. John. "Alleged Psychogenic Disorders in Women—A Possible Manifestation of Sexual Prejudice," *New England Journal of Medicine* (February 1973), 288.

Lévi-Strauss, Claude. *Structural Anthropology*, translated by Claire Jacobsen and Brooke Grundfest Schoepf. New York: Basic Books, 1963.

Levine, Lena, and Doherty, Beka. *The Menopause*. New York: Random House, 1952.

McArthur, Janet W. "Common Menstrual Disorders in the Adolescent Girl," *Clinical Pediatrics*, 3:11 (1964), 663.

McClintock, Martha K. "Menstrual Synchrony and Suppression," *Nature* (London), 229:5282 (1971), 244.

McKinlay, Sonja M., and Jefferys, Margot. "The Menopausal Syndrome," *British Journal of Preventive and Social Medicine*, 28:2 (1974), 108.

McKinlay, Sonja M., and McKinlay, John B. "Selected Studies of the Menopause: An Annotated Bibliography," *Journal of Biosocial Science*, 5 (1973).

MacKinnon, P. C. B., and MacKinnon, I. L. "Hazards of the Menstrual Cycle," *British Medical Journal*, 1 (1956), 555.

Masters, W. H., and Johnson, V. E. *Human Sexual Response*. Boston: Little, Brown and Company, 1966.

Mead, Margaret. *Male and Female*. New York: Dell Publishing Company, 1970.

————. *Sex and Temperament*. New York: William Morrow & Company, 1935.

Michael, R. P. "Determinants of Primate Reproductive Behavior," in *The Use of Non-human Primates in Research on Human Reproduction* (WHO Symposium). *Acta Endocrinologica*, Supplement 166 (1972).

Michael, R. P., and Zumpe, D. "Rhythmic Changes in the Copulatory Frequency of Rhesus Monkeys in Relation to the Menstrual Cycle and a Comparison with the Human Cycle," *Journal of Reproduction and Fertility* (Supplement 10–12), 21 (1970).

Miller, Jean Baker (ed.). *Psychoanalysis and Women*. Baltimore, Md.: Penguin Books, 1973.

Mitchell, Juliet. *Psychoanalysis and Feminism*. New York: Pantheon Books, 1974.

Money, J., and Ehrhardt, A. A. *Man, Woman, Boy, Girl*. Baltimore, Md.: Johns Hopkins University Press, 1972.

Montagu, M. F. Ashley. *The Natural Superiority of Women*. New York: Macmillan, 1953.

————. *The Reproductive Development of the Female with Especial Reference to the Period of Adolescent Sterility*. New York: Julian Press, 1957.

Neugarten, Bernice L., and Kraines, Ruth J. " 'Menopausal Symptoms' in Women of Various Ages," *Psychosomatic Medicine*, 27:3 (1965), 266.

Novak, Emil. *Menstruation and Its Disorders*. New York: D. Appleton & Company, 1921.

O'Connor, J. F., Shelley, E. M., and Stern, Lenore O. "Behavioral Rhythms Related to the Menstrual Cycle," International Institute for the Study of Human Reproduction, New York, 1973.

Oster, Gerald. "Conception and Contraception," *Natural History*, 1972.

Paige, Karen. "Women Learn to Sing the Menstrual Blues," *Psychology Today* (September 1973).

Parlee, Mary Brown. "The Premenstrual Syndrome," *Psychology Bulletin*, 80:6 (December 1973), 454.

Ploss, H. H., Bartles, M., and Bartles, P. *Woman: An Historical, Gynecological and Anthropological Compendium*. E. J. Dingwall (ed.). London: William Heinemann (Medical Books) Ltd., 1935. Published originally as *Das Weib in der Natur-und Volkerkunde*. Berlin: Neufeld & Henius Verlag, 1927.

Pratt, J. P., and Thomas, W. L. "The Endocrine Treatment of Menopausal Phenomena," *Journal of the American Medical Association*, 65 (1937).

Prime Time—For the Liberation of Women in the Prime of Life. Independent feminist monthly, New York.

Rees, L. "The Premenstrual Tension Syndrome and Its Treatment," *British Medical Journal*, 1 (1953).

Ryan, Kenneth J. "Guidelines in Estrogen Therapy," *California Medicine*, 115 (1972), 56.

Scully, Diana, and Bart, Pauline. "A Funny Thing Happened on the Way to the Orifice," *American Journal of Sociology*, 78:4 (January 1973), 1045.

Scully, Virginia. *Treasury of American Indian Herbs*. New York: Crown Publishing Company, 1970.

Seaman, Barbara. *The Doctors' Case Against the Pill*. New York: Avon Books, 1970.

Shader, Richard I., and Ohly, Jane I. "Premenstrual Tension, Femininity and Sexual Drive," *Medical Aspects of Human Sexuality* (April 1970).

Sherfey, Mary Jane. *The Nature and Evolution of Female Sexuality*. New York: Random House, 1972.

Silbergeld, Sam. "The Menstrual Cycle—A Double Blind Study of Symptoms, Mood and Behavior and Biochemical Variables Using Enovid and Placebo," *Psychosomatic Medicine*, 33:5 (1971).

Smith, O. W., and Smith, G. van S. "Menstrual Toxin," in *Menstruation and Its Disorders*, E. T. Engle (ed.). Springfield, Ill.: Charles C Thomas, Publisher, 1950.

Sommer, Barbara. "Menstrual Cycle Changes and Intellectual Performance," *Psychosomatic Medicine*, 34 (1972).

Stevens, William N. "A Cross-cultural Study of Menstrual Taboos," in *Cross-cultural Approaches*, Clellan S. Ford (ed.). New Haven, Conn.: HRAF Press, 1967.

Tanner, J. M. *Growth at Adolescence*. Second edition, Springfield, Ill.: Charles C Thomas, Publisher, 1962.

Thompson, Clara. *On Women*. New York: New American Library, 1971.

Thorne, G. W. "Cyclical Edema," *American Journal of Medicine*, 23 (1957), 507.

Timonen, Sakari, and Procopé, Berndt-Johan. "Premenstrual Syndrome and Physical Exercise," *Acta Obstetrica Gynecologica Scandinavica*, 50 (1971), 333.

Treolar, Alan E., *et al.* "Variations of the Human Menstrual Cycle through Reproductive Life," *International Journal of Fertility*, 12 (1967).

Udry, J. R., and Morris, N. "Distribution of Coitus in the Menstrual Cycle," *Nature* (London), 220 (November 1968), 593.

Wetzel, R. D., and McClure, J. N., Jr. "Suicide and the Menstrual Cycle," *Comprehensive Psychiatry*, 13:4 (1972), 369.

Whalen, Richard E. (ed.). *Hormones and Behavior*. Princeton, N.J.: D. Van Nostrand Company, 1967.

Wilson, Robert A. *Feminine Forever*. New York: M. Evans and Company, 1966.

Women's Health Forum. Series of pamphlets on women's health. Healthright, Inc., 175 Fifth Avenue, Room 1319, New York, New York 10010.

Zacharias, L., and Wurtman, R. J. "Age at Menarche," *New England Journal of Medicine*, 280 (April 1969), 870.

Index

A NOTE ON THE TYPE

This book is set in Electra, a Linotype face designed by W. A. Dwiggins (1880–1956), who was responsible for so much that is good in contemporary book design. Although a great deal of his early work was in advertising and he was the author of the standard volume *Layout in Advertising*, Mr. Dwiggins later devoted his prolific talents to book typography and type design and worked with great distinction in both fields. In addition to his designs for Electra, he created the Metro, Caledonia, and Eldorado series of type faces, as well as a number of experimental cuttings that have never been issued commercially.

Electra cannot be classified as either modern or old-style. It is not based on any historical model, nor does it echo a particular period or style. It avoids the extreme contrast between thick and thin elements that marks most modern faces and attempts to give a feeling of fluidity, power, and speed.

This book was composed, printed, and bound by American Book–Stratford Press, Inc., Saddle Brook, New Jersey.

Typography and binding design by Camilla Filancia